# COGNITIVE BEHAVIORAL THERAPY FOR INSOMNIA

*From Tossing and Turning to Restful Nights*

**ROBERT D. BRADHAM**

Copyright © 2023 by Robert D. Bradham

All intellectual property rights are retained. Without the previous written permission of the author, no part of this book may be reproduced, stored in a retrieval system, or transmitted in any form or by any means, electronic, mechanical, photocopying, recording, or otherwise.

# Table of Contents

**INTRODUCTION** .................................................. 7
Brief Overview of Insomnia ........................................ 7
What This Book Offers ............................................ 11
**CHAPTER 1** ...................................................... 14
**UNDERSTANDING INSOMNIA** ................. 14
Causes And Risk Factors Of Insomnia ................... 20
Effects Of Insomnia On Health And Well Being .... 23
**CHAPTER 2** ...................................................... 29
**CBT FOR INSOMNIA** ................................... 29
Overview Of CBT-I ................................................ 29
Components Of CBT For Insomnia ....................... 32
Evidence Of CBT's Effectiveness In Treating Insomnia .............................................................. 35
**CHAPTER 3** ...................................................... 42
**STIMULUS CONTROL (SCT)** ....................... 42
Explanation Of Stimulus Control Therapy ............. 42

Steps To Implement Stimulus Control Therapy.... 44

Common Obstacles And Solutions..........................52

**CHAPTER 4..................................................62**

**SLEEP RESTRICTION (SRT).....................62**

Explanation Of Sleep Restriction Therapy............ 62

Steps To Implement Sleep Restriction Therapy.... 68

Common Obstacles And Solutions.........................78

**CHAPTER 5...................................................87**

**RELAXATION TECHNIQUES....................87**

Overview Of Relaxation Techniques...................... 87

Instructions For Practicing Relaxation Techniques.. 101

Incorporating Relaxation Techniques Into Daily Routine....................................................................127

**CHAPTER 6................................................141**

**COGNITIVE THERAPY AND RESTRUCTURING.................................... 141**

Explanation Of Cognitive Therapy........................141

Identifying And Challenging Negative Thoughts And Beliefs About Sleep..........................................143

Cognitive Restructuring Techniques And Positive Affirmations..........151

**CHAPTER 7**..........**169**

**MAINTAINING GOOD SLEEP HABITS**.... **169**

Importance Of Good Sleep Hygiene..........169

How To Improve your Sleep Through Sleep Hygiene..........174

Tips For Improving Sleep Environment..........181

**CHAPTER 8**..........**188**

**DEALING WITH SETBACKS**..........**188**

Common Setbacks in the process Of Treating Insomnia With CBT And Solutions..........188

How To Get Back On Track After A Setback..........201

**CHAPTER 9**..........**209**

**CONCLUSION**..........**209**

Recap Of CBT For Insomnia..........209

Encouragement And Final Thoughts..........242

**Sleep Diary**..........**243**

**Glossary of Terms**..........**248**

# INTRODUCTION

## Brief Overview of Insomnia

Insomnia is basically the inability to effectively obtain enough good sleep even when given the chance. Insomnia is a widespread condition whose symptoms might include difficulty falling asleep, remaining asleep, or receiving high-quality sleep (19% to 50% of individuals have reported symptoms in various published surveys). Research on sleeplessness in the developed world's Western states reveals that between 30 and 50 percent of adults claim to experience occasional or mild sleeplessness, and between 10 and 15 percent believe it to be a major issue.

Approximately 35 million Americans report having severe sleeplessness. However, this differs according to age and gender; our 8 to 10-year-olds nearly never complain of sleeplessness, while 25–35% of retirees do.

In general, female prevalence is 1.5 times higher than male prevalence. People who suffer from despair, anxiety, respiratory disorders during sleep, substance addiction, and ongoing health issues are more likely to experience insomnia. It has been said that insomnia is the "common cold" of sleep issues. Just 21% of women and 25% of men claim to have never had insomnia in their lives.

*So, is difficulty sleeping a result of insomnia?*

Yes, but it also affects the person throughout their waking hours. The quality of life is impacted by sleep disorders. This usually manifests as tiredness or a feeling of being depleted, combined with attention issues, focusing, remembering things, and responding quickly.

Insomnia is often claimed to be cognitively and emotionally upsetting, it can result in physiological issues, and can have serious side effects including car accidents and causes interpersonal issues at work, home, school, and other places. Additionally, a lot of people who suffer from chronic insomnia often struggle with depression, anxiety, or are at a higher risk of acquiring these conditions.

## Cognitive Behavioral Therapy and Insomnia

Psychotherapy that focuses on how attitudes, beliefs, and thoughts influence feelings and actions is called cognitive behavioral therapy, or CBT. A person can alter their thoughts, feelings, and behaviors for the better with the use of CBT. It can also give you coping mechanisms to assist you in overcoming obstacles. From chronic pain to depression, cognitive behavioral therapy (CBT) can assist with a wide range of mental health issues. It has a high success rate and is the most recommended therapy for insomnia. It has been demonstrated in recent studies that cognitive behavioral therapy (CBT) is a successful treatment for individuals with chronic insomnia and that it significantly improves sleep diary results.

Using subjective measures, it is seen that these gains in sleep time factors correlate with symptom relief. In a CBT session, you can learn to become conscious of automatic, harmful thought patterns, question underlying presumptions that might be harmful, discern between facts and harmful beliefs, and cultivate a more constructive way of thinking and perceived circumstances. Therefore, changing the ideas, feelings, and actions that contribute to and maintain insomnia is the most efficient and long-lasting treatment for the condition. It has been demonstrated that this method, known as cognitive-behavioral therapy for insomnia, or CBT-I, is more successful than sleeping drugs over the course of several weeks but still outperforms them in the months and years that follow.

## What This Book Offers

A considerable fraction of people suffer from insomnia. Reduced productivity and a worse quality of life may result from its detrimental effects on mental and physical health. Insomnia can be effectively treated without the use of medication by using Cognitive Behavioral Therapy (CBT).

A thorough approach to applying CBT to insomnia treatment is provided in this book. The definition, various forms of insomnia, risk factors, causes, and implications for overall health and wellbeing are all covered in the first chapter. In the Second Chapter, an outline of CBT will be given, along with proof of its efficacy and an examination of its components, which include sleep restriction, relaxation methods, stimulus control, and cognitive therapy.

The particular CBT strategies for insomnia, such as stimulus control, sleep restriction, relaxation techniques, and cognitive therapy, are covered in Chapters Three through Six. Every chapter will provide a detailed explanation of the method as well as step-by-step directions for putting it into practice. We'll also address typical problems and their solutions.

The Seventh Chapter will address the topic of sustaining healthy sleeping practices, including the significance of proper sleep hygiene, suggestions for enhancing the sleeping environment, and methods for adhering to a sleep schedule. We'll talk about typical setbacks and coping mechanisms for setbacks in insomnia treatment in the Eighth Chapter. For individuals wishing to use CBT to cure their insomnia, the Ninth Chapter will offer a summary of the technique as well as some encouragement.

Finally, an appendix will provide a sleep diary for readers to use as they work through the techniques discussed in the book. Overall, this book aims to provide a comprehensive guide to using CBT to treat insomnia, with practical advice and evidence-based techniques.

# CHAPTER 1

# UNDERSTANDING INSOMNIA

## Definition And Types Of Insomnia

Having difficulty falling asleep is a symptom of insomnia, sometimes referred to as *'sleeplessness'*. Those who suffer from insomnia may find it difficult to go asleep, remain asleep, or achieve restful sleep.

The ICSD-3 handbook published by the American Academy of Sleep Medicine defines insomnia as "persistent difficulty with sleep initiation, duration, consolidation, or quality (AASM, 2014)." When you're awake, it has negative effects.

Stress (physical, psychological, or interpersonal) is a common cause of short-term insomnia, which usually lasts for a few days to weeks. Short-term insomnia typically goes away when the stressor is lessened or eliminated, but it can also develop into chronic insomnia, which is characterized by difficulty falling asleep, staying asleep, or waking up early each morning for at least three nights a week for a minimum of three months. Certain actions frequently make chronic insomnia worse. For instance, staying up late in bed in an attempt to sleep more can result in less restful sleep and intervals of waking during the night. Moreover, this may cause irritation, worry, and frustration, all of which have a detrimental effect on sleep quality. Daytime napping, which lessens the demand for sleep at night, and drinking alcohol which has a detrimental impact on sleep quality, both worsen insomnia.

Insomnia can express itself in two ways: sleep-onset insomnia, which refers to trouble falling asleep.

This form of insomnia can occur in persons who have difficulties relaxing in bed, as well as those whose circadian rhythm is disrupted owing to causes such as jet lag or irregular work schedules, and sleep maintenance insomnia, which refers to problems staying asleep after falling asleep. This form of insomnia is frequent among the elderly and those who drink alcohol, caffeine, or smoke before bedtime. Sleep apnea and periodic limb movement disorder can both induce sleep maintenance insomnia. Sleep dissatisfaction is a fourth type of insomnia that is extremely distinct from the others. The complaint here is that you don't feel refreshed even after a seemingly adequate night's sleep.

Many additional forms of insomnia are associated with medical or psychological issues. In such instances, insomnia is considered a comorbidity. Additionally, medicines, illegal drug use, and environmental variables can all have a direct impact on insomnia. However, it is crucial to highlight that insomnia may persist even when the underlying comorbid diseases are resolved. In most situations, both insomnia and the comorbid disease must be addressed in order to alleviate insomnia.

More complicated kinds include pure idiopathic insomnia, psychophysiological insomnia, and paradoxical insomnia, which collectively account for somewhat more than one-third of all insomnia cases. Approximately 15% of all instances of persistent insomnia have no known cause. This is known as primary or idiopathic insomnia. It generally appears early in childhood and can be a lifelong ailment if not addressed. Childhood memories include long, lonely, restless evenings followed by days spent fighting weariness. Many of these persons do not respond well to sleeping medications or stimulants. Although it is thought to be caused by a failure of the brain's sleep/wake systems, rigorous medical evaluation and testing reveal no physical or psychological abnormalities that are causing the insomnia. These persons frequently experience both onset and maintenance sleep issues, and the sleep they do obtain is light and rarely restful. Another 5-7.5% of those diagnosed with insomnia suffer from paradoxical insomnia, also known as sleep state misperceptions. They complain of sleeplessness and may even claim to get no sleep on certain nights. They may describe themselves as light sleepers who notice every slightest sound. They are normally quite concerned about their sleep problems, although they seldom report significant impairment of daytime performance. Despite their concerns, their sleep duration and profile are totally within normal parameters. Some sleep disorder experts believe that paradoxical insomnia exists, but we don't know what to look for or how to assess it. It has been stated that "they think all night long" and that such mental exertion is tiring rather than relaxing. When persons with paradoxical insomnia are treated, their perception of their sleep improves significantly and their worry over it decreases, even though such therapies may have little effect on their actual sleep.

Another 15% of insomniacs experience psychophysiological insomnia. They are frequently persistently hyperactive. When awake, they are agitated, hyperactive, tense, and fearful. It is obvious that such people sleep poorly. Their physiological systems in the brain and body that drive arousal are more intense and lasting. As a result, they are over-aroused, which causes them to be more awake at night and throughout the day. Many have greater levels of arousal hormones and higher body temperatures before bedtime. Psychophysiological insomnia causes people to feel more exhausted than sleepy. They seldom nap, and when they do try, they frequently fail to fall asleep. They do, however, sleep better at the start of their vacation. It's as if they believe they have permission to relax since they're on vacation. Psychophysiological insomnia is typically a chronic disorder that can worsen over time if not managed.

There are less prevalent yet intriguing insomnias, such as temporary insomnia at higher altitudes due to respiratory problems and sleeplessness induced by food allergies. There is also fatal familial insomnia, which is an uncommon but severe illness characterized by increasingly worse insomnia that finally leads to complete inability to sleep within one or many years. People with this disorder have vivid dreams and have a sudden dream-like stupor when they move. It is accompanied by further medical dysfunctions and diseases. It is hereditary.

## Causes And Risk Factors Of Insomnia

More than one-third to one-half of persons seeking medical attention for chronic insomnia have a psychological condition as the major contributor or cause. Both minor and severe psychological issues might have an impact on sleep. People who suffer from anxiety, phobias, or obsessive-compulsive disorder are more likely to have difficulty falling asleep and staying asleep. People with adjustment issues such as ongoing marital or professional stress, as well as those with post-traumatic stress disorder, may have difficulty sleeping. People with schizophrenia, on the other hand, frequently complain about sleep onset issues and poor sleep in general. Several variables are known to have a role in many, if not all, forms of insomnia. One element is the impact of lifestyle. Some people are their own worst enemy when it comes to sleep. For example, people may not practice appropriate sleep hygiene, stay up late on weekends and then sleep the next morning, or take excessive amounts of sleep-inhibiting chemicals. These factors contribute to, and sometimes cause, sleeplessness. It should be clear by now that the causes influencing insomnia are often complicated.

Insomnia risk factors rise with age and may run in families. Shift or night work, noise or light at night, unusually high or low temperatures, and frequent travel to various time zones can all disrupt your sleep-wake cycle, resulting in insomnia. Some negative lifestyle choices, such as excessive alcohol consumption and the use of caffeine and illicit narcotics, lead to insomnia.

Based on the three-factor (3P) model of insomnia, there are three main factors that lead to the development of chronic insomnia: (1) *predisposing factors*, which are characteristics or situations (like high emotional reactivity) that make a person more susceptible to developing insomnia; (2) *precipitating factors*, which are environmental factors (like stressful life events) that cause insomnia to start; and (3) *perpetuating factors*, which are actions and thoughts that help the disorder progress from acute to chronic insomnia and stay long-term.

# Effects Of Insomnia On Health And Well Being

Individuals who suffer from insomnia have the following key characteristics: they have difficulties falling asleep. They lie in bed at the start of the sleep period, longing to sleep but staying awake for a long time. Others can fall asleep easily but struggle to stay asleep all night. Insomnia is defined by a series of relatively protracted waking episodes that interrupt the sleep cycle. Others awaken sooner than wanted; in people with early waking insomnia, sleep onset is relatively quick and sleep continuity is good, but awakening occurs earlier than expected, resulting in insufficient sleep.

Scientists believe this is because lack of sleep alters the hormones that govern appetite and fullness. Long-term sleep deprivation may increase your risk of obesity and the associated health concerns, such as diabetes, high blood pressure, and heart failure.

While you sleep, your body produces proteins that protect you from illness and inflammation. Chronic sleeplessness might disrupt the process. It may also diminish the antibodies and cells that aid your body in fighting illness.
Regular sleep deprivation might impair your body's ability to metabolize blood sugar. This increases your risk of diabetes.

The "brain fog" you experience after a few nights of poor sleep might worsen over time. Chronic insomnia and other sleep problems can impair memory, concentration, and decision-making.

Adults who sleep less than 8 hours a night are more likely to exhibit stress symptoms, such as feeling overwhelmed or losing patience easily, than those who sleep more, according to the American Psychological Association.

Chronic insomnia can eventually cause a mood problem, such as sadness or anxiety.

Fatigue is defined as being so exhausted that it interferes with your professional or personal life, making it difficult to get through the day. It is one of the most prevalent symptoms of persistent insomnia. It is sometimes accompanied by a headache, dizziness, painful or weak muscles.

Finally, Insomnia might reduce your life expectancy.

## *SUMMARY*
## Understanding Insomnia

### Definition
*Insomnia*: Difficulty in falling asleep, staying asleep, or achieving restful sleep. Defined by AASM as persistent difficulty with sleep initiation, duration, consolidation, or quality.

*Short-term insomnia*: Caused by stress, lasting days to weeks. *Chronic insomnia*: Lasts at least three nights a week for a minimum of three months, often exacerbated by certain behaviors.

### Types of insomnia
*Sleep-onset insomnia*: Difficulty falling asleep.
*Sleep maintenance insomnia*: Difficulty staying asleep.
*Sleep dissatisfaction*: Feeling unrefreshed after sleep.

Medical and psychological comorbidities can contribute to insomnia

Complex forms
*Idiopathic insomnia*: No known cause, often lifelong.
*Paradoxical insomnia*: Perception of poor sleep despite normal sleep parameters.
*Psychophysiological insomnia*: Chronic hyperarousal affecting sleep.

## Causes and Risk Factors
*Psychological conditions*: Anxiety, OCD, PTSD, schizophrenia.
*Lifestyle factors*: Poor sleep hygiene, irregular sleep schedules, substance use.
*Risk factors*: Age, family history, shift work, environmental disruptions, lifestyle choices.

Three-factor model (3P)
*Predisposing factors*: Characteristics increasing susceptibility.

*Precipitating factors*: Environmental stressors triggering insomnia.

*Perpetuating factors*: Behaviors and thoughts maintaining insomnia.

**Effects on Health and Well-Being**

Difficulties falling asleep, staying asleep, or waking up too early.

Long-term health risks: Obesity, diabetes, high blood pressure, heart failure.

Immune system disruption and reduced ability to fight illness.

Impaired blood sugar metabolism, increasing diabetes risk.

Cognitive impairments: Memory, concentration, decision-making issues.

Increased stress and risk of mood disorders.

Chronic fatigue impacting daily life.

Reduced life expectancy.

# CHAPTER 2

# CBT FOR INSOMNIA

## Overview Of CBT-I

Cognitive behavioral therapy for insomnia (CBT-i) is an effective non pharmacological treatment that improves sleep outcomes with little side effects and is favored by patients over medication therapy. The approach to CBT-i has evolved in recent years, and it is currently most widely researched as a cognitive and behavioral treatment that includes any or all of five components.

The components will be examined more in following chapters. Furthermore, CBTI outperforms pharmaceutical therapy in terms of retaining treatment improvements after completion. CBT differs from other behavioral therapies in that it includes approaches for altering dysfunctional sleep cognitions.

CBT-I aims to address variables that may contribute to long-term insomnia, such as dysregulation of sleep drive, sleep-related anxiety, and sleep-interfering behaviors. This is performed by using sensory control to develop a learned link between the bed and sleeping, sleep restriction to restore homeostatic regulation of sleep, and cognitive restructuring to change anxious sleep-related thoughts. CBT-I, by modifying sleep-related behaviors and beliefs, may address the variables that cause insomnia to persist. CBT-I is provided in four to eight sessions lasting 30-60 minutes each, either weekly or every other week. There are two major downsides of CBT-I. First, during the first few weeks of therapy, there is generally an acute reduction in total sleep time, which can result in increased daytime drowsiness, which is enough to cause some people to discontinue therapy. Second, benefits from CBT-I are usually not seen until 3-4 weeks into the therapy. While a few studies have looked at the effectiveness of nurse-led CBT-I in primary care settings, in contemporary clinical practice, it is frequently required to refer to people who have specific training in this treatment. It should be emphasized that the main treatments for CBT-I differ significantly from other kinds of CBT, which is why the acronym CBT-I refers solely to this type of CBT for insomnia.

In comparison to medication, treating insomnia with CBT-I offers a number of potential benefits, including less known adverse effects and an intentional focus on addressing the causes that may be responsible for chronic insomnia in order to achieve more long-lasting outcomes. Some patients may prefer non-medicinal therapy. These advantages of CBT-I imply that it might be a more feasible therapy option for insomnia.

## Components Of CBT For Insomnia

Although CBT-I and medication are equally effective in the management of insomnia. CBT-I has been suggested as the first-line treatment because of its long-term effectiveness. CBT-I was designed as a psychological intervention to address the underlying causes of insomnia. It is a short-term, multi-component treatment that combines behavioral and cognitive methods. CBT-I is generally administered over four to eight sessions, with an emphasis on psychoeducation, behavioral, and cognitive methods. Treatments commonly involve stimuli control, sleep restriction, cognitive therapy, sleep hygiene, and relaxation techniques. Each CBT-I component consists of separate skills and methods designed to tackle particular causes of insomnia.

Cognitive Therapy. This tries to discover, question, and change unhealthy ideas and attitudes around sleep and insomnia. Misconceptions about sleep may include unreasonable expectations, dread of losing out on sleep, and an exaggeration of the repercussions of inadequate sleep.

Stimulus control. Behavioral instructions aimed at reinforcing the link between bed and sleep while avoiding the patient from associating bed with other stimulating activitaies. Such recommendations include avoiding nonsleep activities in the bedroom, going to bed only when sleepy, and leaving the bedroom when unable to sleep for 15-20 minutes, then returning to bed only when sleepy.

Sleep restriction. Behavioral recommendations to limit bedtime to match perceived sleep length in order to boost sleep drive and minimize time awake in bed. The time permitted in bed is initially limited to the average amount of sleep perceived every night and subsequently modified to guarantee that sleep efficiency remains more than 85%.

Sleep hygiene. General advice on environmental conditions, physiological aspects, behavior, and routines that support good sleep. Specific recommendations include suggestions on controlling the bedroom environment, such as eliminating visual access to a clock; regular sleep scheduling and avoiding extended daytime naps; and restricting alcohol, caffeine, and nicotine consumption, particularly before bedtime.

Relaxation techniques. Any relaxation method that the patient finds successful can be utilized to lower cognitive alertness and physical tension, allowing for better sleep. Meditation, mindfulness, progressive muscle relaxation, guided imagery, and breathing techniques are among specific strategies that can be applied.

## Evidence Of CBT's Effectiveness In Treating Insomnia

Some studies observed improvements in sleep quality, subjective insomnia severity, drowsiness, psychomotor alertness, mood, anxiety, self-efficacy, sleep-related beliefs and attitudes, health status, and daily function following CBT-I therapy.

Quantitative meta-analyses have indicated that behavioral therapies for sleep are efficacious in children, CBT-i is somewhat effective for anxiety symptoms, and CBT-i is efficacious whether administered in computerized or group-based formats.

Unlike hypnotics, the effects last even after the therapy is stopped. In a direct comparison, CBT-i was found to be more effective than hypnotics for the treatment of persistent insomnia, with benefits lasting 6 months. Furthermore, while hypnotics are an effective therapy for insomnia, their limits include tolerance, side effects, and rebound insomnia following withdrawal.

Because chronic insomnia is a disorder in which almost half of patients remain symptomatic for more than ten years and behavioral therapies are likely to have less side effects therefore CBT-i offers various benefits over pharmacotherapy in this case.

A meta-analysis demonstrates that CBT-i is a very effective treatment for non-comorbid chronic insomnia, providing clinically relevant outcomes. Its effectiveness appears to be long-lasting, with considerable symptom relief. This supports the advice that CBT-i should be utilized as the first line of treatment for persistent insomnia wherever practicable.

Cognitive behavioral therapy for insomnia is helpful, with significant overall benefits on insomnia severity, sleep efficiency, waking time following sleep start, and sleep onset delay. The extent of these improvements is consistent with psychological therapy for other diseases.

Many studies' findings imply that CBT provides much better subjective and objective sleep improvements than no treatment, pharmacological and non-pharmacologic placebo therapies. These studies also indicated that CBT-induced sleep benefits last for 3 to 24 months after therapy. Furthermore, one of these studies found that combining CBT with medication (temazepam) may yield somewhat larger short-term sleep benefits than CBT alone. However, the long-term benefits of this combination strategy are unclear, as many individuals getting this treatment relapse severely over time. In fact, individuals who received CBT alone maintained their sleep gains better than those who received both CBT and medication.

According to meta-analytic estimations, the average treatment effect size is between 1.0 and 1.2, corresponding to a 50% decrease in individual insomnia symptoms following therapy. When total insomnia severity (as measured by the ISI) is taken into account, these treatment effect sizes become significantly larger. Furthermore, the effects of CBT-I are long-lasting, clinical improvements can be sustained for up to 24 months after therapy. Finally, one study found that CBT-I might be useful in treating insomnia in "real world" patients (i.e., those with comorbid medical and behavioral disorders).

## *SUMMARY*
## CBT for Insomnia

**Overview of CBT-I**

Cognitive Behavioral Therapy for Insomnia (CBT-I): Effective non-pharmacological treatment with minimal side effects. Preferred over medication for long-term improvements.

*Components of CBT-I*: Sensory control, sleep restriction, cognitive restructuring.
Aims to address dysregulated sleep drive, sleep-related anxiety, and sleep-interfering behaviors. Typically involves 4-8 sessions of 30-60 minutes. Drawbacks: Initial reduction in sleep time, benefits not seen until 3-4 weeks into therapy.

*Advantages over medication*: Fewer adverse effects, addresses root causes of insomnia.

## Components of CBT-I

*Cognitive Therapy*: Identifies and changes unhealthy thoughts and attitudes about sleep.

*Stimulus Control*: Reinforces the bed-sleep association and avoids stimulating activities in bed.

*Sleep Restriction*: Limits time in bed to improve sleep drive and efficiency.

*Sleep Hygiene*: Provides advice on environmental, physiological, and behavioral factors for good sleep.

*Relaxation Methods*: Techniques to reduce cognitive alertness and physical tension (e.g., meditation, mindfulness).

## Evidence of CBT-I Effectiveness

Improves sleep quality, insomnia severity, mood, anxiety, and daily function.

*Meta-analyses*: Effective for both children and adults, including computerized and group-based formats.

Long-lasting effects compared to hypnotics, with fewer side effects.

More effective than hypnotics for chronic insomnia, with benefits lasting up to 6 months.

CBT-I is recommended as first-line treatment for chronic insomnia.

*Studies*: Significant improvements in sleep efficiency, onset delay, and reduced waking time. Combination with medication may yield short-term benefits, but CBT-I alone maintains long-term gains.

*Meta-analysis*: Average treatment effect size of 1.0 to 1.2, with improvements lasting up to 24 months. Effective for patients with comorbid medical and behavioral disorders.

# CHAPTER 3

# STIMULUS CONTROL (SCT)

## Explanation Of Stimulus Control Therapy

The purpose of stimulus control treatment is to assist people with insomnia in strengthening their bed and bedroom signals for sleep, weakening their bed and bedroom cues for arousal, and creating a regular sleep-wake pattern to support further progress.

Relearning the positive connections of the bed and bedroom with restful sleep is the aim of stimuli control. A number of methods are suggested to do this. These include:

(a) just going to bed when you're tired

(b) establishing a regular wake-up time

(c) getting out of bed and bedroom after extended periods of wakefulness

(d) abstaining from sleep-incompatible activities in bed or the bedroom, such as reading, watching TV, or eating

(e) not taking naps.

The basis of SCT is the theory of behavior and the notion that, depending on the conditioning history, a stimulus can elicit a range of responses. The cues that are often linked to sleep, such as beds and bedrooms, are coupled with excellent sleepers and consequently trigger the sleep response. Those who suffer from insomnia often associate these sleep-related cues with other activities, such as reading, watching TV, or laying in bed and attempting to fall asleep (a practice known as sleep "effort"). Those who engage in these other actions while in bed decrease the likelihood that they will fall asleep at the desired time and location since they are contributing to a maladaptive conditioning pattern, also known as stimulus dyscontrol. As a result, the likelihood that sleep will occur at the desired time and location is reduced. Most significantly, these other acts reinforce the link between one's bed and wakefulness.

## Steps To Implement Stimulus Control Therapy

Stimulus control recommendations include:

(a) lying down to sleep only when sleepy

(b) avoiding using the bed for activities other than sleep or sex

(c) getting out of bed if unable to sleep within 15-20 minutes and returning to bed only when sleepy

(d) repeating this pattern throughout the night as needed

(e) getting up at the same time every day

(f) avoiding napping.

These instructions serve as the foundation for the establishment of healthy sleeping habits and should be followed even after remission has been achieved.

## Common strategies and principles are discussed here

1. *Waking up at a certain time*

Your body utilizes signals such as darkness and brightness to determine when it sleeps and wakes up. Most people who suffer from insomnia sleep longer in the morning to compensate for their late nights. Unfortunately, increasing sleeping hours disrupts your circadian cycle. Waking up at the same time every morning helps enhance your body's sleep signals.

Setting an alarm and getting up at the same time every day enables your circadian rhythm, which governs your bodily signals, to remain consistent. You can set a realistic wake-up time to aid consistency.

This is to develop a steady sleep cycle. This is achieved by establishing a regular wake-up time for all seven days of the week, with no more than an hour of difference between days off and workdays. Irregular schedules are believed to reduce the link between bed and bedroom cues and sleep. Keeping regular sleep habits has been shown to lessen daytime weariness and drowsiness. As a result, maintaining a consistent sleep pattern helps you to reinforce your sleep cues while also reducing daytime difficulties linked with sleep disruption.

2. *Only going to bed when sleepy*

It is normal for a person to go to bed based on the quantity of sleep they believe they require before waking up in the morning. However, this is not the case for people suffering from insomnia, since it merely adds to the stress. After all, sleep occurs when one is calm and pleased. Instead, you should listen to your body and go to bed when you are tired and battling to remain awake.

This instruction is designed to assist you become more conscious of your body's indications for tiredness. Initially, people with insomnia seldom rely on internal indications of drowsiness to tell them when to go to bed. Instead of being seen as a must-begin right now, this step should be seen as an aspirational objective to be accomplished gradually over the first several weeks. You can choose a good time to go to bed depending on your own level of weariness rather than the time on the clock by learning to recognize your own body's sleep signals.

*3. Getting out of bed when not ready to sleep*

This stimulus control strategy is similar to the preceding one. If you realize that you are still awake fifteen minutes after going to bed, get up and go to another room. It might be frustrating for you to lie in bed for an extended period of time without getting any sleep. Though it is difficult to get out of a comfy bed, it will help you become accustomed to the concept that the bed is a place where your mind and body may relax.

When moving to a new room, relax by reading a book or listening to calming music at a low volume. You can then return to bed as you begin to fall asleep and continue this process as many times as necessary.

The instruction to get out of bed if you are not sleeping limits your ability to stay awake in bed and reinforces the relationship between the bed, bedroom, and falling asleep. While SCT is primarily concerned with sleep onset disorders, it has been used to address sleep maintenance concerns too. When unable to sleep, getting out of bed to engage in other activities increases your sense of control over sleeplessness. This alleviates your discomfort and makes the situation more manageable.

*4. Using the bedroom solely for sleeping*

Maintaining the bond between sleep and the bedroom is critical, so use it solely for sleep and relaxation. You should avoid stimulating activities that may keep you awake, such as surfing your phone, watching TV, playing games, eating, or engaging in tense talks.

Furthermore, sleeping anywhere other than the bed undermines the connection between sleep and the bedroom. So, if you start nodding off as nighttime approaches, it's advisable to go to bed. This is meant to reinforce the bed and bedroom cues associated with falling asleep while weakening the cues associated with alertness and wakefulness.

Individuals suffering from insomnia frequently participate in bedtime activities that prevent them from going asleep, such as reading, watching television, playing computer or Internet games, chatting on the phone, texting, checking email, or working. Engaging in these practices creates the bed and bedroom as conditioned triggers for wakefulness rather than sleep. You are to engage in arousal-related activities in another area of the house before entering the bedroom. This will assist you in developing a new nighttime routine that is more suited to facilitating sleep onset.

*5. Avoid napping during the day*

Short naps of 15 to 30 minutes during the day might be a great way to recharge and improve energy and focus. However, this is only true for people who sleep well at night. When using stimuli control treatment, it is best to avoid sleeping throughout the day in order to fall asleep more quickly at night.

This admonition to avoid napping is intended to guarantee that you suffering from insomnia use the previous night's sleep deprivation to help you fall asleep easily the next night. This reinforces the signals of the bed and bedroom for sleep, as well as providing a successful experience for you to sustain compliance with the instructions. It should be noted that we are not against all naps. This is done to enhance the chances that SCT will modify a problematic sleep pattern. Some people, such as the elderly, may benefit from taking a little nap (30 minutes or less) at the same time every day. The irregularity of napping is what causes and maintains irregular sleep habits.

## Common Obstacles And Solutions

*Question*: How long should someone with insomnia stay in bed before getting out if they are unable to fall asleep ?

*Answer*: The guidelines place a high value on getting out of bed fast, often within 10 minutes. However, some people with insomnia feel worried after receiving such advice, and they frequently check the clock to see if it is time to get out of bed. To avoid this clock-checking, you are to move the face of the clock away from you or to keep your watch away from you. If time constraints cause higher concern. This is frequently changed to emphasize the internal indicators of irritation and anguish rather than the amount of time passed. Thus, you are to get out of bed as soon as the first feelings of displeasure at not falling asleep appear. It is crucial to note, however, that staying in bed for extended periods of time while waiting to fall asleep (such as 60 minutes or more) is not permitted, even if not irritated. The purpose of the SCT instructions is to link the bed and bedroom with falling asleep rapidly. According to research, the quarter-hour rule (staying in bed for no more than 15 minutes before falling asleep) is both doable and helpful in improving sleep in people suffering from insomnia.

*Question*: Having gotten out of bed, what activities are permissible, and how long should one stay awake before going back to bed?

*Answer*: A useful clinical rule of thumb for when to return to sleep is that you should be out of bed long enough to feel confident that you will be able to fall asleep if you return to bed. This is a chance to learn noticing internal indications of tiredness and using them as a guide. Generally, this involves staying up for at least 15 minutes or longer before attempting to sleep again. When it comes to what activities are acceptable when you get out of bed in the middle of the night, you should do something peaceful and pleasurable. Because there is growing evidence that even room light may disrupt sleep-wake circadian rhythms, we have placed a greater focus on keeping lights dim when getting out of bed at night. Reading with a reading light is permissible, as is viewing television from a distance. But you are discouraged from doing anything on the computer, even reading email, because the amount of light from the display while sitting near to it is brighter than most people believe, and computer activities are often stimulating.

*Question*: What is the recommended strategy for adults with sleep maintenance problems who wake up early, and how much additional sleep can make a positive impact on alertness and fatigue?

*Answer:* Many adults with sleep maintenance issues prefer to start the day at 4 or 5 a.m. rather than attempting to return to bed for more sleep. This is not a good technique because even an extra

30 or 60 minutes of sleep improves alertness and minimizes weariness throughout the day. As long as the customary final wake-up time is maintained, it is advisable to return to bed when there are 45 minutes or more till wake-up time.

*Notes*

Stimulus control instructions and other behavioral therapies are essentially self-help treatment.

They necessitate active collaboration with you in carrying out tasks. As a result, there is always the issue of people sticking to the treatment plan. Most of the issues related to people compliance with stimulus control recommendations can be resolved by direct conversation with a sleep specialist. When insomniacs get out of bed, they often disrupt their partners' sleep. Discussions about the topic with spouses are frequently beneficial in assuring complete collaboration. Some people in colder areas may be hesitant to leave the comfort of their beds throughout the winter. Solution to this is keeping warm robes beside the beds and an additional room warm throughout the night, along with encouragement to attempt to follow the directions given, all these are typically beneficial in fostering compliance.

## *Summary*
## Stimulus Control Therapy (SCT)

### Explanation of SCT

*Purpose*: Strengthen sleep cues associated with bed/bedroom and establish regular sleep-wake patterns.

*Aim*: Relearn positive connections between bed/bedroom and sleep through methods such as:
Going to bed only when tired.
Establishing a regular wake-up time.
Leaving bed/bedroom after extended wakefulness.
Avoiding non-sleep activities in bed/bedroom.
Not taking naps.

*Theory*: Based on behavioral conditioning; addresses maladaptive conditioning patterns in insomnia patients.

**Steps to Implement SCT**

1. *Lying down only when sleepy*: Enhances awareness of the body's sleep signals. Gradual goal to develop regular sleep habits.

2. *Avoiding bed for activities other than sleep/sex*: Reinforces sleep cues associated with the bed. Prevents a conditioning bed as a place for wakefulness.

3. *Getting out of bed if unable to sleep within 15-20 minutes*: Reduces frustration associated with wakefulness in bed. Encourages engaging in relaxing activities before returning to bed.

4. *Waking up at the same time every day*: Strengthens circadian rhythm.
Minimizes disruption of sleep-wake patterns.

5. *Avoiding napping*: Enhances sleep drive for the night. Reinforces night-time sleep cues.

**Common Strategies and Principles**

1. *Waking up at a certain time*: Consistency in wake-up times improves sleep signals. Regular sleep patterns reduce daytime fatigue and drowsiness.

2. *Going to bed only when sleepy*: Focus on internal sleep signals rather than clock time. Gradually develop awareness of tiredness.

3. *Getting out of bed when not ready to sleep*: Limits wakefulness in bed. Engaging in relaxing activities until feeling sleepy.

4. *Using bedroom solely for sleeping*: Avoid stimulating activities in bed/bedroom. Reinforces the bedroom as a sleep cue.

5. *Avoiding naps during the day*: Increases the likelihood of falling asleep quickly at night. Reinforces sleep pattern regularity.

**Common Obstacles and Solutions**

1. *Time spent in bed before getting out*: Move the clock out of view to avoid clock-watching. Focus on feelings of frustration as a cue to get out of bed. Do not stay in bed for extended periods if unable to sleep.

2. *Permissible activities and duration before returning to bed*: Stay out of bed long enough to feel sleepy. Engage in quiet, enjoyable activities with dim lighting. Avoid computer activities and bright lights.

3. *Waking up early*: Return to bed if 45 minutes or more remain until wake-up time. Even small amounts of additional sleep improve alertness and reduce fatigue.

**Notes**

*Self-help nature*: Requires active participation and adherence to the treatment plan.

*Partner collaboration*: Discuss strategies with partners to ensure cooperation.

*Winter adjustments*: Use warm robes and heated rooms to encourage leaving bed during cold weather.

# CHAPTER 4

# SLEEP RESTRICTION (SRT)

## Explanation Of Sleep Restriction Therapy

A sleeplessness pattern (inability to sleep) might emerge as a result of a stressful or upsetting life event, or as a result of poor sleep practices. This might cause weariness during the day, leading to the assumption that more time in bed is required to make up for lost sleep. However, more time in bed does not result in greater sleep; rather, it results in more time awake feeling anxious or irritated about not being able to sleep. It worsens the condition. Spreading out a night's sleep over an extended length of time will result in shallow and fragmented sleep, resulting in unpleasant moods, increased vigilance at night, and exhaustion throughout the day.

This weariness might be the result of physical strain and mental stress caused by the concern and frustration of insufficient sleep. This cycle of insomnia continues, reinforcing the relationship between the bed setting and attempts to sleep with vigilance and concern. This leads to the development of conditioned insomnia, which is an instinctive reaction to becoming aware in bed. If you completed a Sleep Diary, you undoubtedly discovered that you spend far more time in bed than sleeping.

Can the cycle be changed? **YES!** Spending less time in bed improves your sleep and increases the quantity of deep sleep. What diminishes is shallower, less restorative, light sleep. You will also fall asleep faster, have fewer and shorter nighttime awakenings, and stay asleep until it is time to get up. As a result, you will spend less time worrying about sleep and have more energy during the day.

Sleep Restriction Therapy reduces the amount of time spent in bed, ensuring that sleep happens only between the scheduled bedtime and wake-up time. Your sleep will be of greater quality and last for a shorter amount of time.

Sleep restriction therapy (SRT) is a well-established insomnia treatment that has been utilized in clinical practice for more than 30 years. It is frequently administered as part of multi-component cognitive behavioral therapy (CBT-I).

SRT is recommended for sleep difficulties when the subjective sleep efficiency (sleep time/time in bed - 100%) is less than 85% (or less than 80% in older people). There are also individuals who exhibit relatively high sleep efficiency and yet remain amenable to SRT. For example, there are those who do not get enough sleep on weekdays because they wake up too early. Having learned through experience that if they do resume sleep, it will be right before their alarms ring, they just end the night and get out of bed after, say, 5 hours. However, on non-work days, these people tend to stay in bed long enough to fall asleep again and sleep late into the day. Their sleep efficiency may still be higher than 85% over the course of a week, but such sleepers can benefit from SRT.

SRT starts by calculating three critical sleep features:
(1) average sleep length
(2) daily wake-up time
(3) the part of the night that is likely to include the finest sleep.

These characteristics are best evaluated using a typical 1 to 2 week graphic sleep diary (by averaging estimated total sleep hours and recording daytime wake-up times, as well as examining the patterning of sleep portions within a night).

The TIB (time in bed) at the commencement of therapy is set to the typical sleep length. (The minimum TIB should be 5 hours). The wake-up time on SRT should not be later than the average reported weekday wake-up time. However, the particular bedtime period allotted to each individual will be determined by their sleep pattern. If, for example, a patient's verbal report and sleep log demonstrate that the greatest sleep occurs in the first two-thirds of the night, followed by inconsistent sleep, the assigned wake-up time should be earlier than the average documented workday wake-up time.

For example, suppose an individual reports sleeping 6 hours on average each night out of 8 hours in bed. The initial recommended sleep period is limited to 6 hours. This sleep window is adjusted at regular intervals until the appropriate sleep length is achieved. This causes minor sleep deprivation, which is followed by an increase in sleep duration as efficiency increases.

What is going to happen?
Initially, this management style is difficult to apply. However, the acute sleep restriction during the first several weeks is not permanent. It is used to increase sleep pressure, which helps to ensure better quality sleep in bed and strengthens the bed as a sleep trigger rather than vigilance and concern. By the end of the first week, you should feel more tired, especially before your scheduled bedtime.

Avoid falling asleep before bed (e.g., when watching TV or reading), as this reduces the sleep pressure that should be utilized during the bedtime period. You will most likely feel sleepier than normal when you wake up in the morning and throughout the day. You will need an alarm clock in the morning to guarantee that you do not sleep beyond your specified waking time. It is critical to keep to the new schedule and avoid naps during the day.

Maintaining some 'sleep pressure' from insufficient sleep in the early stages of this strategy can aid your progress. If you stick to the bedtime restriction schedule, it will work and have long-term benefits.

## Steps To Implement Sleep Restriction Therapy

Sleep restriction treatment cannot be administered well unless a thorough sleep journal is available.

Individuals are allotted bedtime hours based on their sleep record, as follows:

Total time in bed (TIB) is equivalent to the individual's assessment of how much sleep he or she gets on average. In no situation should we establish a bedtime of less than 4.5 hours. The time of arising from bed is set to the time the patient usually awakens, and the time of going to bed is determined correspondingly. These designated periods (bedtime to awake time) provide a window for sleep. No napping or sleeping is permitted outside of this window.

An excellent place to start is with the overall amount of sleep time documented in your sleep diary.

This is what you do!

*Step 1*: Determine your average amount of actual sleep every night (using the Sleep Diary, if completed). Make sure you don't add the time you spent laying in bed awake. Plan to stay in bed for only the duration of your determined average sleep time.

For example, the 1-week sleep diary reveals the following:

| Average bedtime to rising time | 10 pm to 5:30 am |
|---|---|
| Average TIB | 7 hrs 30 mins |
| Average sleep latency | 15 minutes |
| Average nightly sleep time | 5 hrs 45 mins |
| Average workday wake-up time | 5:15am |

*Sleep latency is defined as the amount of time between lights out and the time the person actually falls asleep*

The final two hours of sleep are described as "light" and regularly disturbed in the journal.

*Step 2*: Set a regular wake-up time (based on your own circumstances) and adhere to it seven days a week.

*Step 3*: Set a bedtime. To do so, begin with your wake-up time and deduct the amount of sleep hours recorded in your sleep journal. For example, if you want to spend five hours in bed and choose a wake-up time of 6 a.m., your bedtime should be 1 a.m.

You may find it useful to record your intended bedtime restriction schedule.

My average sleep duration will be .............
My bedtime is.............
My wake-up time is ............

The SRT prescription for the initial sleep diary will be as follows

| Allowed TIB | 5 hrs 45 mins |
| --- | --- |
| Bedtime | 11:30 am |
| Wake up time | 5:15 am |

The prescribed TIB, 5 hours and 45 minutes, is based on the computed average nightly sleep time. The choice to get up at 5:15 a.m. was based on reports of bad sleep in the latter two hours of the night.

But assume the sleep latency in the preceding case was 1 hour and 15 minutes, with 30 minutes of arousal following sleep onset normally dispersed in two awakenings. The initial SRT sleep regimen would so be:

| Allowed TIB | 5 hrs 45 mins |
| Bedtime | 12:45 am |
| Wake up time | 6: 30 am |

In this situation, TIB is used later in the night to lessen sleep onset latency. The wake-up time on SRT is set to match the usual weekday wake-up time; working back 5 hours and 45 minutes provided the allotted bedtime.

• 72

Assume the sleep record in the preceding cases shows wakefulness scattered rather evenly throughout the night, with a somewhat lengthy sleep latency of 35 minutes, a couple of awakenings of 15-20 minutes each, and a terminal awakening of roughly 30 minutes. The initial SRT sleep regimen would so be:

| Allowed TIB | 5 hrs 45 mins |
|---|---|
| Bedtime | 12:00 am |
| Wake up time | 5: 45 am |

Now, to address the nightly average of 1 hour and 45 minutes of waking in bed (derived from the sleep log), a later bedtime and an earlier wake-up time are assigned, with the goal of consolidating sleep in between.

You can continue to track sleep on the new schedule and follow-up in one week (7 days).

*Step 4*: Each week, sleep efficiency (SE) is measured using a sleep diary, as per the usual SRT protocol.

If SE is ≥90%, TIB is increased by 15-30 minutes. For elderly persons, the SE cut off for raising TIB is ≥85%.

If SE is 85-90%, TIB remains unchanged. (In elderly adults, the range is between 80 and <85 percent.)

If SE is <85%, TIB is decreased by 15-30 minutes. (In elderly adults, the cut threshold is <80%.)

So, after a week of following the new sleep plan, evaluate how well you sleep. If you're falling asleep faster and sleeping better (SE ≥90) and struggle to remain awake before bedtime, try going to bed 15-30 minutes earlier.

As a general rule, if you are awake in bed for less than 30 minutes (including the time it takes to fall asleep and the time you spend awake during the night), you can increase your overall time in bed.

However, if you are awake for more than 30 minutes (SE <90), do not increase your time in bed yet. Continue with the initial time in bed schedule for another week.

*Sleep efficiency is the percentage of a person's total time in bed that is actually spent sleeping.*

*Step 5*: Maximizing sleep efficiency is not the only goal, since sleep efficiency tends to be best when time in bed is reduced to the recommended minimum of 5 hours but maintaining satisfactory nocturnal sleep and acceptable daytime functioning. At the start of SRT, costs are dramatically increased as well as benefits because significantly less time is spent in bed which is the cost, and vulnerability to really bad nights of sleep is reduced due to an improved homeostatic sleep drive which is the benefit.

However, there's generally a parallel loss in benefits as less sleep is accumulated, resulting in greater tiredness and deficiencies in mood, concentration, and other areas of daily performance. In order to prevent this, after the second week, if you are now having no trouble falling asleep and staying asleep, raise your bedtime by 30 minutes by going to bed 30 minutes earlier.

*Step 6*: The costs and benefits of therapy often rise as it goes on (e.g., less time is spent in bed, but more sleep is acquired). Benefit increases happen more quickly than cost increases do. A maximum net benefit point is attained as the therapy continues. The amount of time spent in bed is limited just enough to preserve a consistent, well-consolidated sleep pattern, but not enough to cause noticeable impairments throughout the day.

This is the goal of the treatment and the timetable that the patient has to make an effort to stick to on their own. Since the majority of the patient's homeostatic sleep need has now been met, there probably wouldn't be much additional benefit in terms of extra sleep if bedtime was increased further, possibly to its baseline value. However, there would be a higher risk of reintroducing variable, interrupted sleep.

In simpler terms
Continue with the Step 5 schedule until you feel you are receiving appropriate sleep (i.e., you are less drowsy and weary) and your sleep is still of excellent quality (less than 30 minutes of waking time in bed). If, however, you discover that excessive wakefulness in bed has returned, you have prolonged your bedtime too long and too rapidly. Reduce your bed period again by going to bed 30 minutes later and repeat Step 4. Once you've found your optimum bedtime and sleep schedule, stick to it. Consider the extra time obtained by lowering your overall time in bed to be a positive consequence. Use your newly acquired free time in a productive or entertaining manner.

## Common Obstacles And Solutions

*Question*: Do I have to be in bed trying to sleep at the scheduled bedtime?

*Answer*: We don't demand that you do this. However, you are still needed to get out of bed in the morning at the appointed hour, even if you remain out late on the weekends. We emphasize that the main purpose of the schedule is to prevent you from napping or being in bed outside your bedtime to wake-up time. You are also not allowed to lie down after the designated bedtimes.

*Question*: How can I ensure compliance with sleep restriction therapy, and what flexibility do I have in setting my sleep schedule while still following the therapy's guidelines?

*Answer*: Compliance is a key concern with sleep restriction therapy, as it usually is with behavioral therapies. As a result, even while we are clear on the overall structure of the therapy, we work together to choose the specifics. After determining what the starting schedule should be, based on the sleep log, ask if you can live with the bedtimes. Changes to the timetable can be made by you if they do not contradict the spirit of the process. However, you are advised that if the timetable does not suit you, you should not just modify it on your own. Any changes to the regimen can be considered by both you and a sleep doctor in order to prevent making rash, ill-conceived decisions.

*Question*: How can I manage the side effects of SRT?

*Answer*: Some people may be extremely sensitive to the negative effects of SRT and so find the restrictions excessively tough. Intolerance might manifest as weariness, drowsiness, memory impairment, irritability, or decreased focus over a short period of time. Despite the possibility of increased sleep depth and efficiency at the onset of SRT, this intolerance of daytime deficiencies may prevent adherence to SRT for long enough to consolidate improvements. One change to the SRT technique that accounts for this is to set the starting TIB equal to the reported average amount of sleep plus 30 minutes. This is a reasonable and moderate adjustment to SRT that eases the individual into a restricted bedtime schedule.

*Question*: How do you stay alert during sleep restriction therapy?

*Answer*: It's not unusual to feel drowsy during the day. Adjusting to SRT might take some time, and you may feel tired than normal at first. If so, stimulate your brain by putting on bright lights, exercising or going on a stroll, and staying away from "comfortable" places like a sofa or bed before bedtime. Avoid using stimulants such as coffee or energy drinks, as these might disrupt your sleep routine as well.

**Notes**

SRT enhanced sleep propensity (particularly at the onset of therapy) will cause sleepiness. Individuals who require constant alertness to avoid major accidents should not participate in SRT. Long-haul truck drivers, long-distance bus drivers, air traffic controllers, heavy machinery operators, and some assembly-line workers, for example, would be put at an unacceptable danger as a result of SRT-induced drowsiness. Similarly, people who have disorders that are aggravated by sleepiness or deep sleep, such as epilepsy, parasomnias, and sleep disordered breathing, should avoid SRT.

Individuals who fall asleep fast and experience brief, compact sleep prior to a fatal early morning waking (even on non-workdays and vacations) are unlikely to benefit from SRT. In these instances, limiting time in bed will not (1) improve sleep latency, (2) reduce the frequency or length of awakenings, and (3) is unlikely to increase sleep duration.

When people describe staying in bed "completely awake" only to rest, judgment must be used. The capacity to perceive sleep is poor (sometimes to a large degree, as in paradoxical insomnia, formerly known as sleep-state misperception), and people may be unaware that they are obtaining some sleep after the primary sleep phase. In circumstances where some light or unappreciated sleep occurs at the end of the night, SRT may be useful.

## *SUMMARY*
## Sleep Restriction Therapy (SRT)

### Concept and Benefits of SRT
Stress or poor sleep habits can lead to insomnia, causing daytime fatigue and a misconception that more time in bed is needed.

More time in bed often results in more awake time, leading to anxiety and worsening sleep quality.

SRT limits time in bed to improve sleep quality, increase deep sleep, reduce sleep latency, and decrease nighttime awakenings.

SRT is a part of Cognitive Behavioral Therapy for Insomnia (CBT-I) and has been in use for over 30 years.

### Indications for SRT
SRT is recommended for sleep efficiency below 85% (or 80% in older adults).

SRT can benefit individuals with inconsistent sleep patterns even if their overall sleep efficiency is above 85%.

**Steps to Implement SRT**

1. *Evaluate Sleep Patterns*: Use a sleep diary to determine average sleep length, wake-up time, and best sleep period.

2. *Set Time in Bed (TIB)*: Initially, TIB is set to average sleep length (minimum of 5 hours), with a fixed wake-up time.

3. *Weekly Adjustment*: Adjust TIB based on sleep efficiency (SE) measured weekly:
   - SE ≥90%: Increase TIB by 15-30 minutes.
   - SE 85-90%: Keep TIB unchanged.
   - SE <85%: Decrease TIB by 15-30 minutes.

4. *Consistency*: Maintain strict bedtime and wake-up times, avoid naps, and adhere to the schedule to build sleep pressure.

5. *Monitor and Adjust*: Continue adjustments until optimal sleep duration and quality are achieved.

## Common Obstacles and Solutions

*Scheduled Bedtime*: Flexibility is allowed, but the wake-up time must be adhered to.

*Compliance*: Collaborate with a sleep doctor to tailor the schedule.

*Managing Side Effects*: Start with a slightly longer TIB if experiencing severe side effects.

*Staying Alert*: Use bright lights, exercise, and avoid stimulants.

## Precautions

SRT is not suitable for individuals requiring constant alertness, or those with certain medical conditions like epilepsy or sleep-disordered breathing.

It is less effective for individuals with naturally compact sleep or those staying in bed "completely awake."

By following these steps and guidelines, SRT aims to consolidate sleep, improve sleep quality, and reduce daytime fatigue.

# CHAPTER 5

# RELAXATION TECHNIQUES

## Overview Of Relaxation Techniques

Relaxation therapy, which has long been used to treat insomnia, entails treatments that address physiological and cognitive arousal in the context of sleep-related performance anxiety and nighttime arousal. The therapy's purpose is to diminish or remove sleep-disrupting physiological factors such as muscular tension and cognitive arousal, such as racing thoughts.

*Progressive muscle relaxation, autogenic training, biofeedback-assisted relaxation, guided imagery training, deep breathing exercises, physical activity, meditation, and hypnosis* are examples of formal relaxation approaches. Regardless of the approach used, this therapy includes learning and practicing relaxation techniques.

Here's a overview of the several relaxation techniques:

**Progressive Muscle Relaxation**

*Progressive muscular relaxation* can be used simultaneously with deep breathing or guided visualization exercises. The method is also known as Jacobson's Relaxation. The method entails tightening and releasing different muscle groups to induce sensations of peace and relaxation.

Beginning with your feet, gently tighten your muscles for 5 to 10 seconds before swiftly releasing, noting the sensation of tension melting away. Repeat with your other muscles, progressing upward through your body until you reach your scalp. This is a rather physical approach, therefore users must avoid overworking or straining their muscles. It is also critical to take deep, steady breaths while performing the steps. You may need to practice progressive muscle relaxation for a few weeks before getting the hang of it and starting to see effects.

Progressive muscular relaxation consists of seven phases.

*Step 1*: Select a room with few distractions and sit or lie comfortably.

*Step 2*: Contract the muscles in the foot for 5 seconds before releasing the contraction for 10 seconds. Focusing on releasing tension and feeling the muscles relax helps promote tranquility. To avoid leg cramps, spread your toes rather than curling them.

*Step 3*: Contract and release the muscles in your lower legs for the same length of time.

*Step 4*: Repeat with the hips and buttocks.

*Step 5*: Next, focus on the muscles in your stomach and chest.

*Step 6*: After exercising the torso, contract and release your shoulders.

*Step 7*: The facial muscles come next. You can contract your face by pressing your eyes shut for 5 seconds and then releasing for 10 seconds.

## Autogenic Training

*Autogenic Training* is a strategy that can promote psychological and physical serenity. It entails slowing and regulating one's breathing while also educating the body to respond to vocal commands.

During practice, you concentrate on the physical feelings of various sections of your body, particularly warmth, heaviness, and relaxation.

Some people will need the help of a professional practitioner, while others prefer to do it themselves.

## Biofeedback-Assisted Relaxation

This approach uses electrical instruments to monitor several body processes, such as skin temperature, heart rate, and muscular tension. Its goal is to assist a person regulate or relax a certain region of their body.

The treatment entails attaching sensors to a specific portion of the body and taking measurements as the subject relaxes. A user may then utilize the input to assist them make changes as needed, such as relaxing a specific muscle.

Although most biofeedback-assisted relaxation is performed in specialized therapy facilities, certain portable equipment is available for purchase. However, before acquiring these items, you should consult with a healthcare expert to determine that they are safe for usage.

## Guided Imagery Training

Everyone has a happy place - a location where they feel wonderful. Perhaps it's your favorite beach, a lakeside seat, or a sun-dappled woodland route.

When you're feeling stressed, try shutting your eyes and envisioning this environment. Take a few seconds to mentally scan these lovely surroundings and recollect the peaceful feeling of being there.

The more you practice, the easier it will be to mentally transport yourself to your happy spot.

Many people utilize this approach to relax and focus themselves during stressful situations.

*Guided imagery* replaces negative or stressful sensations with pleasant and peaceful experiences. Some people may prefer the aid of a healthcare professional or a recording, whilst others opt to practice by themselves.

Guided imagery has three steps:

*Step 1*: Sit or lie down in a comfortable position. Ideally, find an area with low distractions.

*Step 2*: Imagine a tranquil atmosphere by recalling one from memory or creating a new one. Consider environmental factors through the five senses: sight, hearing, smell, taste, and touch.

*Step 3*: Continue the visualization for as long as necessary, taking slow, deep breaths and focusing on peaceful emotions.

**Deep Breathing Exercises**

Deep Breathing is linked to a slower heart rate and lower blood pressure, according to specialists. When you inhale, your belly expands but not your chest. This indicates that you are breathing deeply. This explains why deep breathing is often known as belly breathing.

To practice, sit in a comfortable chair and breathe deeply ten times. Keep one hand on your tummy and feel it expand with each breath. Breathing exercises make people feel more calm.

Deep breathing entails taking slow, deep, even breaths. Box breathing is a breathing technique that some individuals find beneficial, and most people do not need expert assistance.

Box breathing has four easy steps:

*Step 1*: Breathe in through your nose for 2-4 seconds.

*Step 2*: Then, hold your breath for 2-4 seconds.

*Step 3*: Breathe out for 2-4 seconds.

*Step 4*: Finally, hold your breath for another count of 2-4 seconds. Repeat as required.

## Physical Activity

It may seem unusual, but moving your body might help you relax. According to the Anxiety & Depression Association of America, physical activity causes the production of endorphins, or "feel-good" chemicals, which promotes sleep. Even a single 30-minute session of moderate-to-vigorous exercise, such as brisk walking, may alleviate anxious feelings.

The Centers for Disease Control and Prevention (CDC) suggest 150 minutes of physical exercise each week for best health.

Some kinds of exercise also incorporate features of mindfulness. This is the discipline of paying attentive attention to the current moment without passing judgment, as well as to your own breathing patterns.

These exercises include the following:

*Tai chi or Qigong*. This low-impact workout involves moving slowly and steadily through a sequence of motions that replicate animal gestures, such as a bird extending its wings. The emphasis is on being aware of your breath and body sensations as you progress through the various positions.

*Yoga*. There are several types of yoga that you may study through online tutorials or live classes. Some are slower-paced, while others are more active. One common aim of all yoga practices is to breathe deeply and steadily as you progress through the various postures, or asanas.

## Meditation

Meditation may improve your sleep. As a relaxation method, it may calm the mind and body while promoting inner peace. Meditation, when practiced before bedtime, can help alleviate insomnia and sleep problems by boosting general tranquility.

When you meditate, you experience a number of physiological changes. These changes induce sleep by influencing various bodily systems.

For example, in a 2015 study published in JAMA Internal Medicine, researchers looked at how mindfulness meditation influenced 49 persons who had moderate sleep problems. Participants were randomly allocated to 6 weeks of meditation or sleep hygiene education. At the conclusion of the trial, the meditation group had less insomnia symptoms and less daytime weariness.

Meditation, according to the experts, appears to be beneficial in a variety of ways. Stress and worry are common causes of sleep disorders, but meditation might help you relax more effectively. It also enhances autonomic nervous system regulation, reducing the ease with which you are woken.

Meditation may also :
- Increase melatonin (the sleep hormone).
- Increase serotonin (a precursor to melatonin).
- Reduce cardiac rate.
- Lower blood pressure.
- Engage areas of the brain that regulate sleep.

Your body undergoes comparable adjustments in the early stages of sleep. As a consequence, meditation can help you sleep by triggering these adjustments.

Meditation has several advantages, including improved sleep. When practiced frequently, meditation can also:
- Improve your mood.
- Reduce stress.
- Reduce anxiety, boost attention, and improve cognitive function.
- Reduce tobacco cravings.

- Improve your pain response and lower high blood pressure.
- Improve cardiovascular health
- Reduce inflammation

**Hypnosis**

According to The Sleep Charity in the United Kingdom, sleep hypnosis can assist some people fall asleep if they are struggling with insomnia. However, it may not be effective for persons who are not susceptible to hypnosis, and it seldom works as a standalone therapy.

Hypnosis can sometimes help with insomnia because it helps people let go of their worry. A meta-analysis published in 2019 looked at the efficacy of hypnosis as an anxiety therapy. The researchers discovered that it was more successful when paired with other psychological therapies.

## Benefits of Relaxation Techniques

Doctors advise that relaxing may aid persons who are managing a range of various health issues, such as:

- Labor pain.
- Heart illness.
- Chemotherapy-related nausea
- Chronic pain.
- Temporomandibular Joint Pain

It is crucial to note that relaxation techniques take practice before they become effective, so don't expect them to work right away.

# Instructions For Practicing Relaxation Techniques

**BREATHING TECHNIQUES**

The 4-7-8 breathing may help you gain control over your breathing. It involves inhaling for 4 seconds, holding your breath for 7 seconds, and exhaling for 8 seconds. The 4-7-8 technique forces the mind and body to focus on regulating the breath, rather than replaying your worries when you lie down at night. Proponents claim it can soothe a racing heart or calm frazzled nerves.

The overall concept of 4-7-8 breathing can be compared to practices like:

Alternate nostril breathing entails breathing in and out of one nostril at a time while holding the other nose closed.

Mindfulness meditation facilitates focused breathing while bringing your attention to the present moment.

Visualization concentrates your thoughts on the course and pattern of your natural breathing.

Guided imagery helps you focus on a positive memory or tale to alleviate stress while breathing.

People who are having modest sleep difficulties, anxiety, or tension may find that 4-7-8 breathing helps them overcome distractions and relax.

Proponents of 4-7-8 breathing claim that with regular practice, it grows increasingly powerful. According to reports, the effects are not immediately obvious. You may feel a little lightheaded the first time you try it. Practicing 4-7-8 breathing at least twice a day may produce better outcomes for certain people than those who just practice once.

## How To Do It

To practice 4-7-8 breathing, locate a comfortable spot to sit or lie down. It is important to exercise appropriate posture, especially when starting off. If you're utilizing the method to fall asleep, laying down is ideal.

Prepare for the exercise by placing the tip of your tongue on the roof of your mouth, directly below your top front teeth. You will need to maintain your tongue in place during the practice. It takes discipline to avoid moving your tongue when you exhale. Some people find it simpler to exhale during 4-7-8 breathing when they purse their lips.

The following stages should be completed in a single breath cycle:

- First, let your lips part. Make a whooshing sound and exhale entirely through your lips.

- Close your lips and inhale discreetly through your nose while counting to four in your thoughts.

- Then hold your breath for seven seconds.

- Take another eight-second exhale with whooshing motion.

- When you inhale again, a new breathing cycle begins. Repeat this sequence for four full breaths.

The most important aspect of this technique is to hold your breath for seven seconds. It is also advised that you just practice 4-7-8 breathing for four breaths when you initially begin. You can progressively build up to eight full breaths.

This breathing method should not be used in situations if you are not ready to totally relax. While it is not often used to fall asleep, it can induce deep relaxation in the practitioner. Make sure you don't need to be completely awake right after practicing your breathing cycles.

## AUTOGENIC TRAINING

Autogenic training is a relaxing method that focuses on instilling sensations of peace and relaxation in your body to assist reduce stress and anxiety.

### How To Do It

Autogenic training is most effective when done with a skilled practitioner, such as a therapist. Once you're familiar with the process, you may start using these relaxation techniques on your own.

Here are the steps utilized in autogenic training to lower stress and alleviate anxiety symptoms.

- Set up. Before you start, choose a peaceful, comfortable area to relax. Ideally, you should practice relaxation methods in the same location each time.

- You may perform these exercises lying down or sitting up. Take care to take off your glasses and adjust any tight clothes.

- Begin with your breath. The first step is to calm your breathing. Make sure you're in a comfortable posture and begin with calm, even breathing.

- Once you've regulated your breathing, remind yourself, "I am completely calm." Saying this to oneself may be enough to induce a sense of calm.

- Pay attention to different portions of your body.

- Start with your right arm and repeat the statement, "My right arm is heavy, but I am completely calm," while breathing slowly and steadily.

- Repeat this with your other arm and legs, constantly returning to "I am completely calm."

- Pay attention to your heartbeat.

- While inhaling deeply, tell yourself six times, "My heartbeat is calm and regular," and then, "I am completely calm."

- This continues for other parts of your body, such as the belly, chest, and forehead.

In addition to these procedures, you may choose to use a voice recording with instructions. This helps you to completely relax and focus on the technique.

## GUIDED IMAGERY

Guided imagery is a technique for dealing with stress. It is a relaxing method that entails imagining nice, serene environments such as a lovely beach or a tranquil meadow. This approach is sometimes called visualization or guided meditation.

Anxiety and worry can make it difficult to sleep comfortably. However, some research suggests that guided imagery may help you sleep better.

Participants in a 2017 study reported improved sleep after using guided imagery.

Similarly, a 2015 research of older persons discovered that a mindfulness practice using guided imagery may have the potential to enhance sleep quality. The researchers hypothesized that mindfulness meditation improves your body's response to stress, making it easier to sleep.

## What are your requirements to get started

Guided imagery may be done at any time and from any location, with no need for specific equipment. In general, you'll need:

- A peaceful and quiet location and a comfy couch, bed, or yoga mat.

- A guided imagery audio recording is optional.

- Headphones (Optional)

- Guided imagery audio recordings are accessible on numerous platforms, such as: YouTube (search for "guided imagery"), Headspace app, Simply Being App.

- Your local bookstore or library may also carry guided imagery CDs.

**How To Do It**

Follow these step-by-step instructions to practice guided imagery without using an audio recording:

- Sit or lie down in a calm, pleasant environment.

- Close your eyes. Take several deep breaths.

- Inhale and exhale deeply, and maintain breathing deeply as you repeat this relaxation exercise.

- Consider a serene landscape, such as a verdant forest, a stunning mountain range, or a quiet tropical beach.

- Consider a favorite area in nature that helps you feel comfortable.

- Consider the details in the scenario.

- Consider the sounds, fragrances, and sensations of being in this serene, tranquil environment.

- Imagine a walkway in your setting.

- Imagine yourself traveling along the route, taking in the details and noises.

- Take a few minutes to relax in your environment.

- Continue to breathe deeply.

- After fifteen minutes, count to three. Open your eyes.

If you're new to guided imagery, these tips may be useful:

1. You may read a script or listen to an audio recording. It is advised that you listen to a recording and close your eyes while performing this exercise.
2. Choose a peaceful spot where you won't be bothered.
3. Wear comfortable, relaxed clothes.
4. Turn off your phone and other devices. Set your phone's recording mode to "do not disturb."
5. Take several deep breaths. Take a deep breath in and out before beginning the audio recording.

6. Continue to take deep inhalations and exhalations while following the audio recording's recommendations.

7. Don't be concerned about how well you are doing.
8. Relax, don't strive too hard, and allow the process to unfold naturally.

Guided imagery requires practice. Start with 5 minutes every day and gradually increase the time.

If you're having trouble envisioning serene situations, search for photographs or movies on the Internet. Find a relaxing setting and believe you are there.

Keep a record of how you feel after using guided imagery. You may measure your stress levels over time to see if they've improved.

## PROGRESSIVE MUSCLE RELAXATION

Edmund Jacobson, an American physician, established PMR in the 1920s. It was founded on the idea that physical relaxation might aid in mental calm.

Jacobson discovered that you can relax a muscle by tensing and then releasing it. He also noticed that doing so helps to calm the mind.

PMR offers a foundation for obtaining this level of relaxation. It requires you to focus on one muscle group at a time. This helps you to identify the stress in that particular place.

It's also important to tighten each muscle group before relaxing. This motion heightens the sensation of relaxation in the region.

PMR is a simple approach to do at home. You do not require any extra equipment or gear. All you need is focus, attention, and a peaceful location where you will not be disturbed.

The key to this method is to tense and hold each muscle group for 5 seconds. Then you exhale and allow your muscles to completely relax for 10 to 20 seconds before moving on to the next muscle group.

**How To Do It**

- Begin by laying or sitting down. Relax your whole body. Take five deep and steady breaths.

- Lift your toes high. Hold and then release. Pull your toes down. Hold and then release.

- Next, strain your calf muscles, then relax.

- Bend your knees toward each other. Hold and then release go.

- Squeeze your thigh muscles. Hold and then release go.

- Clench your hands. Pause and then let go.

- Tense your arms. Hold and then release

- Squeeze your buttocks. Pause and then let go.

- Contract the abdominal muscles. Pause and then let go.

- Contract the abdominal muscles. Pause and then let go.

- Inhale and tighten your chest. Hold, exhale, and release.

- Raise your shoulders towards your ears. Pause and then let go.

- Purse your lips together. Hold and then release.

- Open your mouth wide. Hold and then release.

- Close your eyes tightly. Pause, then release.

- Raise your eyebrows. Hold and then release.

**Tips for Beginners**

If you're new to relaxation methods or PMR, consider the following helpful tips:

1. Set about 15-20 minutes for PMR. Do it in a calm, comfortable environment.

2. Turn your phone off to avoid distractions.

3. Avoid holding your breath, which can increase tension. When you tension your

muscles, take a deep breath in and exhale fully.

4. Move in a pattern that works for you. For example, you can start at your head and work your way down your body.

5. Wear loose, light clothes.

6. Practice PMR even when you are feeling calm, especially at first. This will make it easy to understand the process.

## BIOFEEDBACK THERAPY

Biofeedback therapy is a non-drug treatment in which patients learn to regulate body processes that are generally automatic, such as muscular tension, blood pressure, or heart rate.

As it is noninvasive and does not require medicines, there is a reduced possibility of unwanted side effects.

There are three common forms of biofeedback treatment.

1. *Thermal biofeedback* monitors skin temperature.

2. *Electromyography is used* to monitor muscular tension.

3. The goal of *neurofeedback*, also known as *EEG biofeedback*, is to regulate electrical brain activity.

During a biofeedback session, the therapist applies electrodes to your skin, which transmit data to a monitoring box.

The therapist examines the measures on the monitor and, via trial and error, determines a variety of mental exercises and relaxation techniques that can aid in the regulation of your body processes.

You then eventually learn how to manage these processes yourself, eliminating the need for monitoring.

## MEDITATION

Meditation is a simple activity that may be done anywhere and anytime. You do not require any special tools or equipment. In truth, you simply need a few minutes.

However, developing a meditation regimen requires practice. Making time for meditation increases your chances of reaping the advantages.

Here are the fundamental stages for meditation:

1. Find a calm place. Sit or lie down, whichever seems most comfortable. It is recommended to lie down at nighttime.

2. Close your eyes and take calm breaths. Inhale and exhale deeply.

3. Concentrate on your breathing. If a thought arises, let it go and concentrate on your breathing.

Be gentle with yourself when trying meditation for sleep. A meditation practice is exactly that, a practice. Begin by meditating for three to five minutes before bedtime. Over time, gradually extend the duration to 15 to 20 minutes. Learning to calm your thoughts will take time.

Let's have a look at some particular meditation techniques that work well for sleep and how to use them.

## Mindfulness Meditation

Mindfulness meditation entails focusing on the present. It works by raising your awareness of your consciousness, breathing, and bodily responses and if you notice a thought or feeling while in practice, just observe it and let it go without judging yourself.

How to practice mindfulness meditation

- Remove all distractions from your room, including your phone.

- Lie in a comfortable position.

- Concentrate on your breathing. Inhale for 10 counts, followed by 10 counts of holding your breath. Exhale for ten counts. Repeat five times.

- Inhale and stiffen your body. Pause, relax, and exhale. Repeat five times.

- Pay attention to your breath and body. If a bodily part is tense, intentionally relax it.

- When a thought comes up, steadily redirect your concentration to only your breathing.

## Guided Meditation

Guided meditation is when another person takes you through each phase of meditation. They may tell you to breathe or relax your body in a specific way. Alternatively, they can ask you to picture images or sounds.

At bedtime, consider listening to a guided meditation audio recording.

Here's where you'll discover recordings:

Meditation resources include podcasts, apps, websites, internet streaming services (such as Spotify), and local libraries. While the specific methods may differ from one source to the next, the step-by-step directions below offer a basic overview of how to practice guided meditation.

## How to Do Guided Meditation
- Choose a recording.
- Dim the light on your phone or device while listening to the guided meditation.
- Start the recording. Lie down in bed and take long, steady breaths.
- Concentrate on the person's voice. If your thoughts stray, gradually restore your focus on the recording.

## Body Scan Meditation

Body scan meditation involves focusing on each component of your body. The purpose is to raise your awareness of physical feelings, such as tension and discomfort. The process of focussing encourages relaxation, which can aid in sleep.

## How to Practice Body Scan Meditation

- Remove all distractions from your room, including your phone. Lie in a comfortable position.
- Close your eyes and take calm breaths.
- Consider the weight of your body on the bed.
- Concentrate on your face. Relax your jaw, eyes, and face muscles.
- Move to your neck and shoulders. Relax them.
- Continue down your body, focusing on your arms and fingers.
- Continue with your stomach, back, hips, legs, and feet. Consider how each portion feels.

If your thoughts stray, gradually return your awareness to your body. If you like, you can go in the reverse direction, from your feet to your head.

## HYPNOSIS

Hypnosis for insomnia entails relaxing and entering a trance-like condition to relieve anxiety. This may result in their spending more time in deep sleep, which is essential for healing and memory storage.

People can try self-hypnosis, which is comparable to meditation. Alternatively, they might consult a hypnotherapist, but hypnosis only works if the individual wants it.

First, there is a conversation about the person's goals for the session and an agreement on the hypnosis approaches the therapist will utilize.

Next, the hypnotherapist:
Encourages deep relaxation and employs agreed-upon approaches to achieve goals. Gently lifts the person out of their trance-like condition, leaving them feeling rejuvenated and calm.
When hypnotized, the subject is completely in control and is under no obligation to accept the

hypnotherapist's instructions. They also have the option of waking up from the hypnotic condition.

## Incorporating Relaxation Techniques Into Daily Routine

In order to get consistent and long-term insomnia treatment, you must include relaxing methods into your everyday practice. Meditation, progressive muscle relaxation, and deep breathing can all help you maintain a sense of calm and balance, which is essential for good sleep.

*Schedule Relaxation Time*: Make self-care a priority by setting aside specified periods for activities like meditation or deep breathing. By prioritizing relaxation as a daily activity, you guarantee that you regularly make time for stress-reduction activities and encourage better sleep.

*Choose a Suitable Technique*: Look for the relaxation techniques that you love and start with it. Incorporating relaxation techniques you enjoy into your regular routine makes relaxing a normal part of your day. You can also mix and match approaches based on your mood to make your activities interesting and fun, allowing you to unwind and enhance your sleep quality.

*Start small:* Choose one or two relaxation techniques that appeal to you, such as deep breathing or meditation. You add them into your regular routine and do it for a few minutes each day, this way you avoid overburdening yourself and establish a consistent practice that promotes relaxation and decreases stress, which can assist with insomnia.

*Create a Calming Environment*: Design a peaceful spot in your house for relaxing. To create an attractive atmosphere, include soft lighting, comfy seats, and relaxing scents. This way you will have a go-to spot for relaxing and practicing relaxation techniques, which may help to calm your mind and body before bedtime. Having a designated tranquil environment will help you easily incorporate relaxation into your daily routine.

*Unplug Periodically*: Set aside certain times in your day to disconnect from electronic devices and participate in relaxation-promoting activities such as nature walks or mindfulness practice. Including these unplugged minutes in your routine allows you to disengage from stresses and focus on relaxing activities, which improves your capacity to relax and fall asleep more quickly.

*Practice Mindfulness*: Incorporate mindfulness into your regular and relaxation activities by becoming completely present in the moment. Whether at work or at home, taking a few deep breaths and concentrating on the present moment can help to decrease tension and relax. Regular mindfulness practice throughout the day promotes a more relaxed mentality, which can contribute to better sleep.

*Prioritize relaxation*: Make relaxing daily priority to maintain your health and well-being. Incorporate relaxation methods into your daily routine to improve your mood, reduce stress, and increase your general feeling of well-being. Recognizing the value of relaxing, will help you stay dedicated to practicing relaxation techniques and manage insomnia more successfully.

*Relaxation with Others:* Include social components in your relaxation schedule by inviting friends or family to join you in relaxation activities or exchanging suggestions and experiences. This social component may make your relaxation activities more fun and give additional support, allowing you to remain motivated and consistent in your practice.

*Write It Down*: Keep a journal to record your relaxation activities and ideas. Writing down your experiences reinforces your practice and serves as a helpful tool for self-reflection. Regular journaling will help you measure your progress, recognize stress reductions, and stay dedicated to adopting relaxing techniques into your everyday life.

By using these steps, you may establish a long-term habit that promotes relaxation and helps with insomnia. Each step is intended to smoothly include relaxation methods, making them an essential part of your routine and promoting quality sleep.

*SUMMARY*

Relaxation Techniques

**Overview of Relaxation Techniques**

Relaxation therapy, historically utilized to treat insomnia, addresses physiological and cognitive arousal in sleep-related performance anxiety and nighttime arousal. Its goal is to reduce or eliminate sleep-disrupting factors such as muscular tension and racing thoughts. Techniques include progressive muscle relaxation, autogenic training, biofeedback-assisted relaxation, guided imagery, deep breathing exercises, physical activity, meditation, and hypnosis. This chapter provides an overview of these techniques and instructions on how to practice them.

**Progressive Muscle Relaxation**

Overview: Also known as Jacobson's Relaxation, this method involves tightening and then releasing different muscle groups to promote relaxation.

**Steps**:

1. *Preparation*: Select a distraction-free room and sit or lie comfortably.

2. *Feet*: Contract foot muscles for 5 seconds, release for 10 seconds.

3. *Lower Legs*: Contract and release muscles in the lower legs.

4. *Hips and Buttocks*: Repeat the process.

5. *Torso*: Focus on stomach and chest muscles.

6. *Shoulders*: Contract and release shoulder muscles.

7. *Face*: Contract facial muscles by pressing eyes shut, then release.

**Autogenic Training**

Overview: This technique promotes psychological and physical calm by controlling breathing and responding to verbal commands to focus on body sensations like warmth and heaviness.

**How To Do It:**

1. *Setup*: Find a quiet, comfortable place to relax.
2. *Breath Focus*: Begin with calm, even breathing.
3. *Body Focus*: Sequentially focus on different body parts, repeating calming statements.
4. *Heartbeat Focus*: Inhale deeply, affirm a calm heartbeat, and relax.

**Biofeedback-Assisted Relaxation**

Overview: Uses electrical instruments to monitor body processes like skin temperature, heart rate, and muscle tension to help control these areas.

**How It Works**

1. Monitoring: Sensors are attached to the body, providing data on physiological processes.
2. Feedback: Use the data to adjust and relax specific body areas.

**Guided Imagery Training**

Overview: Involves visualizing peaceful settings to replace negative or stressful feelings with positive and calming experiences.

Steps

1. *Setup*: Sit or lie down comfortably in a distraction-free area.
2. *Visualization*: Imagine a tranquil environment using all five senses.
3. *Relaxation*: Continue the visualization while taking deep breaths.

**Deep Breathing Exercises**

Overview: Linked to slower heart rates and lower blood pressure, deep breathing, or belly breathing, promotes calmness.

**Box Breathing Technique**

1. *Inhale*: Breathe in through your nose for 2-4 seconds.
2. *Hold*: Hold your breath for 2-4 seconds.

3. *Exhale*: Breathe out for 2-4 seconds.
4. *Hold*: Hold your breath again for 2-4 seconds.
5. *Repeat*: Continue as needed.

**Physical Activity**

Overview: Exercise promotes the release of endorphins, enhancing sleep. Activities like tai chi, qigong, and yoga incorporate mindfulness and promote relaxation.

**Meditation**

Overview: Meditation calms the mind and body, promoting inner peace and alleviating insomnia by reducing stress and anxiety.

**Benefits**

- Increases melatonin and serotonin levels.
- Reduces heart rate and blood pressure.
- Engages brain areas regulating sleep.

**Hypnosis**

Overview:Sleep hypnosis can assist those with insomnia by promoting relaxation and reducing anxiety. It is often more effective when combined with other psychological therapies.

**How It Works:**

*Preparation*: Relaxation and entering a trance-like state.

*Goals*: Setting goals with a hypnotherapist and following their guidance.

Benefits of Relaxation Techniques

Relaxation techniques can help manage various health issues, including labor pain, heart disease, chemotherapy-related nausea, chronic pain, and temporomandibular joint pain.

## Instructions for Practicing Relaxation Techniques

Breathing Techniques: 4-7-8 Breathing

1. *Preparation*: Find a comfortable spot, sit or lie down, and maintain good posture.

2. *Breath Cycle*:
   - Exhale completely through your mouth.
   - Inhale quietly through your nose for 4 seconds.
   - Hold your breath for 7 seconds.
   - Exhale completely through your mouth for 8 seconds.

3. *Repeat*: Continue for four full breaths.

Autogenic Training

1. *Setup*: Choose a quiet place, sit or lie comfortably, remove distractions.

2. *Breathing*: Start with calm, even breathing.

3. *Body Focus*: Sequentially focus on different body parts, repeating calming statements.

Guided Imagery

1. *Setup*: Sit or lie down comfortably in a quiet place.
2. *Visualization*: Imagine a peaceful scene using all senses.
3. *Relaxation*: Continue visualization with deep breaths.

Progressive Muscle Relaxation

1. *Preparation*: Lay or sit down, relax your body.
2. *Muscle Tensing and Relaxing*: Focus on one muscle group at a time, tensing for 5 seconds, then relaxing for 10-20 seconds.

Biofeedback Therapy

1. *Monitoring*: Use sensors to monitor physiological processes.
2. *Adjustments*: Use feedback to learn how to control and relax specific body areas.

Meditation

1. *Setup*: Find a quiet place, sit or lie down.
2. *Breathing*: Take calm, deep breaths.
3. *Focus*: Concentrate on your breathing and let go of distracting thoughts.

Incorporating these relaxation techniques into your daily routine can help manage stress and improve sleep quality. Start with one or two techniques and practice them consistently to see the best results.

# CHAPTER 6

# COGNITIVE THERAPY AND RESTRUCTURING

## Explanation Of Cognitive Therapy

Cognitive therapy aims to change sleep-related cognitions (e.g., beliefs, attitudes, expectancies, and attributions) that are thought to contribute to the persistence or worsening of insomnia.

The primary idea of this strategy is to examine negative feelings (fear, anxiety) that sleeplessness might bring forth that are incompatible with sleep.

For example, if a person is unable to sleep at night and begins to dwell on the potential consequences of sleep deprivation on the following day's performance, this can set off a chain reaction that feeds into the vicious cycle of insomnia, emotional distress, and more sleep disturbances.

Within this conceptual framework, cognitive therapy is designed to guide you in identifying some unhelpful sleep-related cognitions and beliefs and reframing them with more adaptive substitutes in order to short-circuit the self-fulfilling nature of this vicious cycle.

The process of cognitive restructuring includes recognizing and addressing problematic ideas. As an example, you can assist individuals feel differently about things that bother or annoy them.

Cognitive restructuring strategies may also be used in everyday life to help people manage stress, advance in their careers, or sleep better. It takes no professional training, however a psychotherapist can assist you in mastering the skills.

The purpose of cognitive restructuring is to foster balanced and realistic thinking, rather than to make a person think favorably. It can help a person think differently about a variety of subjects, including: Relationship issues, poor self-esteem, sadness, anxiety, sleeplessness, and stress.

## Identifying And Challenging Negative Thoughts And Beliefs About Sleep

Specific therapeutic objectives include (but are not limited to):

- unreasonable expectations regarding sleep requirements ("I must get my 8 hours of sleep every night").

- incorrect assumptions regarding the causes of insomnia ("My insomnia is entirely due to a biochemical imbalance");

- excessive stress about sleep loss and its implications ("Insomnia will have serious consequences on my health"),

- as well as misunderstandings about appropriate sleep habits ("If I only try harder, I'll eventually return to sleep").

Cognitive therapy for unhelpful sleep-related beliefs employs the same clinical procedures (e.g., reappraisal, reattribution, decatastrophizing, attention shifting, hypothesis testing) as cognitive management of other disorders such as anxiety and depression. Cognitive approaches such as Socratic questioning, collaborative empiricism, and guided discovery allow you to:

(1) identify your unfavorable automatic beliefs regarding sleep and insomnia that are speculated to prolong the target problem;

(2) detect the links between cognitions, emotions, and behaviors.

(3) Consider the facts for and against your sleep-related distorted automatic ideas.

(4) Replace these biased cognitions with more accurate interpretations, and

(5) Learn to recognize and adjust their basic beliefs that lead to inaccurate impressions of the situation.

So, how do you do all this?

One is self-monitoring, which is often a very successful method for identifying automatic thinking. It may be accomplished through the use of Socratic verbal questionings and picture recollection.

For example, if you're having difficulties sleeping, you may train your mind to recognize your habitual thoughts and feelings.

You may do this by asking questions such as, "What was on your mind when you couldn't sleep last night?", "How did you feel at the time?", and "What did you think then?" Home practice is extremely crucial in cognitive treatment.

The automatic thoughts record form is a highly valuable evaluation tool to monitor a wider variety of dysfunctional thoughts than those reported during therapy sessions. It is also a practical tool to assist you continue monitoring your sleep-related unpleasant automatic thoughts.

# Example of a Standard Three-column Automatic Thoughts Record Form

| Situation<br><br>**Specify Date and Time** | Automatic Thoughts<br><br>**What was Going Through Your Mind?** | Emotions<br><br>**Rate Each Emotion's Intensity on a Scale of 1–100%** |
|---|---|---|
| 04/28: Checking emails at 8pm | I must sleep well tonight<br><br>I have so much work tomorrow | Anxious (50%) |
| 04/29: Lying in bed awake at 2 am | This has to stop! I can't go on living like this.<br><br>This is going to make me ill. I have to get some sleep | Anxious (75%)<br>Discouraged/sad (60%) |

Once you've recognized your sleep cognitions and are familiar with thought-monitoring, the next stage is to consider your thoughts as just one of many possible interpretation. The next step in therapy is to find alternatives to dysfunctional sleep cognitions by employing cognitive restructuring techniques to weaken the association between sleeplessness and the negative thoughts that are hypothesized to maintain the aroused state. To help oneself evaluate the validity and usefulness of your cognitions, ask probing questions like:

What evidence supports this idea?
What is the evidence against?
Why do you believe this will happen? What are the possibilities of this happening? What is the worst thing that might happen?
Could you survive it?
Are there any different perspectives on this situation?
What is the most realistic scenario?

The next step in therapy is to find alternatives to dysfunctional sleep cognitions by employing cognitive restructuring techniques to weaken the association between sleeplessness and the negative thoughts that are hypothesized to maintain the aroused state.

Self-monitoring is still incredibly essential at this point in order to adjust your perspective on sleep and recognize how much your emotional reaction varies depending on the nature of the ideas you entertain. To that end, two columns are added to the three-column automatic ideas form: a fourth column where you can indicate probable alternative ways of perceiving things (i.e., more sensible and realistic views).

For example, finding evidence for and against the thought/belief, listing the impact of the thought on your emotions, or estimating the likelihood that the feared outcome will occur; and a fifth column in which the associated emotions are reassessed in light of this alternative thinking.

| Situation<br><br>Specify Date and Time | Automatic Thoughts<br><br>What was Going Through My Mind? | Emotions<br><br>Rate each Emotions Intensity on a Scale of 1–100% | Alternative Thoughts<br><br>How Can I See This Situation Differently? | Emotions<br><br>Rate Each Emotions Intensity on a Scale of 1–100% |
|---|---|---|---|---|
| 04/08: Wide awake at 2am | Not again! I definitely won't be able to function at work again | Anxious (90%) | There is really no point in worrying about this right now. I can't force sleep anyway I can usually still get some work done after a poor night sleep, worrying will only make things worse and keep me awake even longer. | Anxious (15%) |

## Cognitive Restructuring Techniques And Positive Affirmations

You may identify the cognitive distortions that are harming you by using cognitive restructuring strategies. They can help clarify the reasons behind illogical or incorrect thinking. Additionally, it might teach you how to "question" negative thinking patterns and replace them with more constructive ones.

Here's a brief guide to some of the strategies involved in cognitive restructuring:

**Self-Monitoring**
To recognize the counterproductive thought processes that keep you up at night in order to stop the cycle of insomnia is critical. Although cognitive restructuring is a potent technique, its effectiveness depends on your capacity to identify the ideas that set off your insomnia.

You may get ready for those times and stop these ideas in their tracks by becoming aware of the places and times when they occur. If, for example, you frequently find yourself worrying about things like "I'll never fall asleep, I'll be exhausted tomorrow, and my entire day will be ruined," you can be reinforcing a catastrophizing behavior. You may catch these ideas and recast them in a more positive way by recognizing this pattern.

Writing in a journal might be a useful tool for this process. Even if you don't know what's causing your insomnia, journaling your thoughts can help you find faulty thought patterns and pinpoint areas that need attention. You'll become more aware of these tendencies and more capable of confronting them as you practice self-monitoring, which will open the door to a good night's sleep.

**Challenging Your Assumptions**

Learning to challenge your beliefs and assumptions is a crucial component of cognitive restructuring, particularly when those beliefs appear to stand in the way of leading a fruitful life.

It's simple to become engrossed in unfavorable ideas and thoughts while you're having trouble falling asleep. You can learn from a therapist how to investigate these ideas and identify prejudices and nonsensical thinking by applying Socratic questioning techniques.

Here are some inquiries you may pose to yourself:

Are these thoughts supported by evidence or is it just my concern?

What proof do I have for this thoughts being true?

What proof exists that this thoughts might not be true?

How can I verify the accuracy of these thoughts through testing?

What might go wrong if I don't get a restful night's sleep?

How can I get ready for and handle that scenario?

Any other alternative perspectives on this matter that wouldn't keep me up at night?

Are things actually this bad, or are there any gray areas?

For example, you may believe that you will always be tired or that you will never be able to go asleep if you find yourself worrying excessively about getting enough sleep. By challenging this way of thinking, you might set a task for yourself to make a list of every scenario that could happen and then assess the likelihood of each one. This might assist you in thinking through fresh options that aren't as extreme as the ones that keep you up at night."

**Gathering Evidence**

Acquiring evidence is an essential phase in cognitive restructuring, particularly in the context of treating insomnia. By keeping track of your events, feelings, and thoughts, you may start to confront the unfavorable patterns that keep you up at night.

Think about maintaining a journal or sleep diary to record:

The things or people you were with and what you were doing right before bedtime.

The intensity of your reactions (such as how nervous or scared you feel).

Any recollections or ideas that cross your mind when you're lying awake. Additionally, compile information supporting or refuting your theories, assumptions, and opinions regarding sleep.

As an illustration:

Make a note of the occasions you have gone to sleep and had restful sleep if you think you will never be able to do so. If you think you're the only one who has trouble sleeping, find out the prevalence of insomnia by looking up data. If you believe that you will always be tired, monitor your energy levels and make a note of the moments when you feel relaxed and focused.

By gathering information and conducting an unbiased analysis of it, you may start to question your cognitive distortions and swap them out for more sensible, well-rounded ideas. You may break the cycle of insomnia and develop sound sleeping habits by doing this.

**Carrying Out A Cost-Benefit Evaluation**

To assess the benefits and drawbacks of clinging to unfavorable ideas and opinions about sleep, do a cost-benefit analysis.

Consider this:

- What good does it do me to believe "I'm a failure for not sleeping well" or "I'll never fall asleep"?

- What are the costs of these views, both practically and emotionally? (For instance, heightened worry, exhaustion, and reduced productivity)

- How will this affect my physical and mental health in the long run?

- What impact do these ideas have on my interpersonal relationships? (As in, agitation, retreat)

- How do they affect my performance on a daily basis and my capacity to meet objectives?

You may make an informed decision about whether it's worthwhile to challenge and alter these thought patterns by weighing the advantages and disadvantages side by side. This can assist you in cultivating a more positive and balanced thinking, which will enhance your general wellbeing and quality of sleep."

**Generating Alternatives**

You may confront your negative thought patterns that keep you awake and discover new ways to think about sleep with the aid of cognitive restructuring. Creating logical replacements for the distortions and alternate explanations is a part of this process.

As an illustration:

- Consider other possibilities, such as "I'm feeling anxious tonight, but I've fallen asleep in tough situations before," rather than thinking, "I'll never fall asleep."

- Rather than thinking, "I'll be exhausted forever," you can think, "I've had difficult days before and I can do it again."

- You might come up with alternatives like "I've prepared well for tomorrow" or "I can tackle challenges as they come" if you can't sleep at night fretting about what has to be done tomorrow.

Creating empowering affirmations to counteract false or ineffective beliefs is another aspect of generating alternatives.

You might say this to yourself again:

- "I've overcome sleep struggles before and can do it again."
- "I'm capable of relaxing and falling asleep."

- "I've made progress and can continue to improve my sleep."

You may start to change your perspective and establish a more positive relationship with sleep by coming up with alternatives and repeating encouraging statements.

Positive phrases repeated on a regular basis to replace negative and sometimes false beliefs are known as affirmations, according to neuroscientist Chelsie Rohrscheib, Ph.D., who specializes in sleep and mental health.
Affirmations can help you establish reasonable expectations for the next night and stop negative thoughts in their tracks when you use them before bed.

Affirmations are a sort of meditation as well. Research published in the Journal of Sleep Health indicates that even in those without pre-existing sleep issues, several forms of meditation can help reduce insomnia and enhance the quality of one's sleep. Meditation reduces breathing and heart rate, which are physiological indicators that your body's autonomic nervous system which regulates unconscious physiological reactions has transitioned from "fight or flight" to "rest and digest." Additionally, studies that were published in the journal show that it reduces cortisol levels, which is a stress hormone.

According to Rohrscheib, expecting a bad night's sleep might make it worse. "That's because when we expect to sleep poorly, we get more stressed and anxious.

And as stress levels rise, we are more prone to have insomnia, mid-sleep awakenings, and less time spent in the deep, restorative stages of sleep.

Sleep affirmations, on the other hand, can lower tension, put you in a better frame of mind for sleep, and help you sleep better. They can also help you stick to a nightly routine, which is the gold standard of good sleep hygiene.

"Our brains thrive on routines and patterns, and this is especially true when it comes to sleep," Rohrscheib states. "Following a consistent pre-bedtime routine is one of the best ways to signal to the brain it's time for sleep."

There is no one-mantra-fits-all sleep affirmation; for the best results, choose the one that feels appropriate to you.

Make it about **YOU**. "Affirmations should be tailored to your specific circumstance," Rohrscheib argues. "For instance, if the main reason you're having trouble falling asleep is that you keep thinking of the stressors you encounter at work, you might come up with affirmations that help you reframe how you think about those stressors: 'I choose to release my work stress' or 'I can control how my work affects me.'"

Concentrate on the now. Instead of placing conditions like "I will relax when it's time to go to sleep," Rohrscheib suggests keeping your affirmations in the present tense.

Keep it light. This is the time to tap into your inner positivism and realism.

Not sure where to start? Rohrscheib recommends these sleep affirmations (but feel free to tailor them to make them unique to you ! : )

"I will sleep soundly all through the night."
"I will enjoy deep, restorative sleep tonight."
"My bedroom is a place of relaxation and deep sleep."
"In my bedroom, my thoughts naturally detach and slow down."
"I will get up as soon as my alarm goes off and feel fresh and alert."

If you are experiencing racing thoughts due to certain situations, you can also try:

"Right now the answer to my problems is restful sleep."
"I am opening my mind to peace and that is where I will find sleep."
"Tonight I am following my heartbeat, towards a good night's sleep."
"I am grateful for today and this night, where I am going to get my rest."
"I deserve to sleep tonight so I am refreshed for tomorrow."

*SUMMARY*

## Cognitive Therapy and Restructuring

**Explanation of Cognitive Therapy**

Aims to change sleep-related cognitions (beliefs, attitudes, expectancies) contributing to insomnia. Focuses on examining negative feelings that interfere with sleep. Guides individuals in identifying and reframing unhelpful sleep-related beliefs.

**Identifying and Challenging Negative Thoughts and Beliefs about Sleep**

*Specific therapeutic objectives*:

Unreasonable expectations regarding sleep ("I must get 8 hours every night").

Incorrect assumptions about insomnia causes ("It's entirely due to a biochemical imbalance").

Excessive stress about sleep loss consequences ("Insomnia will have serious health effects").

Misunderstandings about sleep habits ("If I try harder, I'll fall asleep").

*Techniques used*:
Socratic questioning, collaborative empiricism, and guided discovery.
Identifying automatic beliefs, linking cognitions to emotions and behaviors, and replacing distorted thoughts with accurate interpretations.

**Self-Monitoring**
Important for recognizing automatic thinking patterns. Can be achieved through Socratic questioning and using an automatic thoughts record form.

**Cognitive Restructuring Techniques**
*Self-Monitoring*: Recognize and record counterproductive thoughts.

*Challenging Assumptions*: Use Socratic questioning to investigate and challenge negative thoughts.

*Gathering Evidence*: Keep a journal or sleep diary to record events, emotions, and thoughts.

*Cost-Benefit Evaluation*: Assess the practical and emotional costs and benefits of clinging to negative thoughts.

*Generating Alternatives*: Develop logical replacements for cognitive distortions and create empowering affirmations.

**Positive Affirmations**

Replace negative beliefs with positive, constructive statements.

*Examples*:
  - "I will sleep soundly all through the night."
  - "My bedroom is a place of relaxation and deep sleep."
  - "I will get up as soon as my alarm goes off and feel fresh and alert."

- Tailor affirmations to your specific situation and keep them in the present tense.

**Benefits of Affirmations**
- Reduce stress and anxiety.
- Improve sleep quality.
- Promote a consistent pre-bedtime routine.

# CHAPTER 7

# MAINTAINING GOOD SLEEP HABITS

## Importance Of Good Sleep Hygiene

If you rely on an alarm to get up, hit snooze many times, feel drowsy while driving, rely on caffeine or energy drinks, lack attention, and make basic blunders, experience forgetfulness as sleep deprivation affects short term memory. Sleep deprivation can cause depression, anxiety, and irritability. It can also impair the immune system, leading to recurrent diseases.

If you are experiencing any of these symptoms, you most likely have bad sleeping habits. However, we can help you modify this by optimizing your sleep hygiene.

**But what are the poor habits that impair your sleep?**

*Drinking Alcohol*: Alcohol is a sedative that can put you to sleep quickly. However, it metabolizes in your system over a few hours, causing sleep disturbance and poor sleep quality. Drinking alcohol can also dehydrate you and produce grogginess or a hangover, reducing your capacity to wake up refreshed.

*Long Daytime Napping*: This one may be a bit controversial. Some cultures encourage midday naps, and many individuals swear by them. If you sleep well at night, it may not be an issue. However, if you are having difficulty sleeping, the last thing you want to do is add gasoline to the fire by napping during the day. Naps impair your capacity to sleep at night, and severe daytime drowsiness might indicate a sleep condition such as sleep apnea.

*Taking Caffeine and Smoking Cigarettes*: Caffeinated beverages such as coffee, tea, soda pop, and foods such as chocolate act as stimulants, keeping you alert for hours. Caffeine should be avoided between 4 and 6 hours before bedtime, or earlier if you are sensitive to its effects. Similarly, the nicotine in a cigarette can impair your ability to sleep, and the yearning associated with withdrawal may wake you up during the night.

*Lying Awake in Bed*: If you're having difficulties falling asleep, the last thing you should do is lie awake. If this happens on a regular basis, as it often does with insomnia, you may come to associate your bed with worry and a lack of sleep. Instead of tossing and turning, engage in a soothing activity such as reading. If you're still having trouble sleeping, get out of bed. This can also occur when you utilize your bed for purposes other than sleep or sex.

*Changing Your Sleep Time From One Day to the Next*: We are creatures of habit, and our sleep is no different. If you go to bed and wake up at various times every day, your body will lose track of when it should feel weary and drowsy. This is ultimately determined by our natural clock, known as the circadian rhythm, and changing our sleep schedules can have a severe impact on it. We can sleep better when we stick to a set schedule. Begin by setting an alarm for your waking time and going to bed when you feel drowsy, ensuring that you receive adequate sleep on a consistent basis.

*Eating a Large Meal Before Bedtime*: Nothing beats a full bladder or stomach to interrupt your sleep. Getting up to pee disrupts restful sleep, so drinking too much before bed may result in frequent trips to the bathroom during the night. Eating a heavy meal close to bedtime may cause heartburn symptoms when you lie down, which can be painful. Obstructive sleep apnea can also induce nocturia and heartburn throughout the night.

## *What you enjoy when you keep a good sleep hygiene*

Sleep hygiene refers to a set of practices that promote good quality sleep. These include lifestyle and nutritional practices that are consistent with the body's natural cycles.

Some individuals define excellent sleep hygiene as sticking to a regular sleep schedule and avoiding consuming alcohol before going to bed. These and other habits can aid with sleep quality and general well-being.

Long-term, poor sleep hygiene can lead to sleep problems such as insomnia, whereas excellent sleep hygiene can provide you with the following advantages below and more:

Increased daytime energy
Improved mood
Improved immune system function.
Reduced stress
Improved cognitive function
Improved blood glucose control
Improved mental health which leads to increased productivity and a higher overall quality of life.

## How To Improve your Sleep Through Sleep Hygiene

**Have a sleep routine**
The body runs on a 24-hour internal clock. This influences how it works, including how it controls your temperature and mood. Developing a regular sleep-wake cycle helps to regulate the body's clock.

To do this, consider getting up at the same time every day, including on weekends and holidays.

Then, schedule a bedtime that allows you at least 7 hours of sleep every night.

However, it is advisable to avoid going to bed without feeling drowsy and staying awake in bed.

**Avoid certain foods and beverages before bedtime**

Caffeine and nicotine are stimulants that can keep the body awake, so avoid taking them at least 4-6 hours before bedtime.

Coffee, tea, cola and chocolates should be avoided before bedtime. Cigarettes, and some drugs, such as those for colds, flu, and migraines, are all potential sources of caffeine or nicotine.

Also, avoid alcohol 4-6 hours before bedtime because it might have a detrimental impact on sleep quality.

**Create an environment that promotes sleep**
Keeping the bedroom cold might aid with sleep. According to the National Sleep Foundation, a temperature of 60-67°F is optimal. If light or noise are a concern, consider using blackout shades or wearing an eye mask or earplugs. Some people find that white noise, such as that produced by a fan, helps.

To assist reinforce the brain relationship between the bed and sleep, limit bedroom activities to sex and sleeping.

It might also be beneficial to invest in a comfortable mattress and bedding that promotes spinal alignment and helps regulate body temperature.

**Relax before bedtime**
Creating a calming routine to decompress before bed helps the body recognize that it is time to sleep.

Avoid screens, such as phones and computers, for at least 1-2 hours before bedtime. The blue light from these devices can interfere with the generation of melatonin, a hormone that regulates sleep.

A relaxing routine might include listening to soothing music, reading something not too stimulating, or engaging in another soft activity.

Taking a warm bath or shower 1-2 hours before bedtime might also help you relax. Furthermore, when the body cools after a shower or bath, the reduction in temperature might stimulate sleep.

**Get up if you're not sleeping**
If you haven't fallen asleep after 20 minutes, get out of bed. Sit somewhere dark and quiet, and engage in a relaxing, non-stimulating activity. When you become drowsy, you might return to bed.

**Refrain from sleeping with pets**

You may consider your pet to be a member of the family, so why not share your bed with them? 45 percent of Americans let their pets sleep on their beds, yet this might be the source of your insomnia. Many individuals have allergies to cats and dogs, which can be increased by sharing a bed. These allergens can stay in clothing, pillows, and mattresses, potentially causing a response. With so many different types of pet beds and crates to choose from such as a nesting bed, raised bed, or heated bed it may be time to seek an alternative resting arrangement for your buddy.

**Avoid taking naps so close to the evening**

Short power naps are recommended and beneficial, but extended naps in the late afternoon and evening might have a detrimental impact on your sleep quality. Instead, keep naps to 15 to 30 minutes in the early afternoon. This increases your chances of waking up feeling revitalized while also making it easier to fall asleep at nighttime. Your circadian clock slows in the early afternoon between 2pm and 3pm which might make you feel drowsy and in need of a nap. This is the finest time to fall asleep without disturbing your sleep at night.

**Exercise regularly to have better sleep**

Exercise not only produces endorphins, but it also helps you fall asleep faster and wake up feeling refreshed. Even just 10 minutes of exercise at any time of the day can significantly improve sleep quality. Getting a decent sweat may be accomplished by joining a local gym, meeting with a personal trainer on a regular basis, or choosing a physical activity that you love. If you have a limited schedule, you may even set up an in-home gym for flexibility and convenience.

**Avoid snoozing the alarm**

You actually wake up tired after snoozing your alarm, especially if using the snooze button several times is part of your pattern. You can't get to a restorative level of sleep between alarms, which confuses your brain and disrupts the natural wake-up process. If you sleep seven to nine hours per night, your body shouldn't require any further sleep and may even begin waking up on its own before your first alarm goes off. Reduce the amount of times you snooze the alarm clock until you can wake up after only one.

**Other tips:**
The following methods can also assist enhance the quality and consistency of sleep.

- Get some natural light when you get up in the morning.

- Avoid monitoring the time at night, since this may induce or worsen your worry about sleep.

- Even if you are fatigued, try to keep up with your everyday activities, unless it is unsafe.

- Avoid eating 2-3 hours before bedtime.

- Avoid intense exercise four hours before bedtime.

- Stay hydrated during the evening, but don't drink too much before bed to minimize overnight visits to the bathroom.

## Tips For Improving Sleep Environment

It is essential to make the bedroom a relaxing environment for sleeping. You can do this by:

Maintaining a cool environment, keep the temperature between 60°F and 70°F. Remove any items that create noise or light. Use blackout curtains to guarantee adequate darkness. Remove debris off the bed and tidy the space surrounding it. Use smooth bed sheets and coverings.

To prepare for sleep, make sure pillows are properly positioned, off bright lights, close blinds, and turn on a bedside lamp or night light, and cool the room by adjusting air conditioning, opening a window, or using a fan.

Daytime light exposure is advantageous, however nocturnal light exposure has the reverse impact.

Again, this is due to its influence on your circadian cycle, which tricks your brain into believing it is still daytime. This decreases secretion of hormones such as melatonin, which aid in relaxation and deep sleep.

Blue light, which is produced in abundance by electronic devices such as cellphones and laptops, is the most harmful in this respect.

There are numerous strategies for reducing nocturnal blue light exposure. This includes:

- Wear glasses that block blue light.

- Install a blue light-blocking app on your laptop and smartphone. These are accessible for both iPhone and Android devices.

- Stop watching television and turn off any bright lights two hours before going to bed.

Set an alarm one hour before you want to go to bed to remind you to put down your gadgets and start your evening routine or read instead

Declutter your space. Keeping your bedroom neat and free of unwanted distractions is vital for your body to begin to relax. Important job paperwork, busy artwork, or even a treadmill are all irritating reminders of your duties that might keep you awake while you try to sleep. Instead, keep your bedroom clutter-free and the decor to a minimum.

.

## SUMMARY
## Importance of Good Sleep Hygiene

*Signs of poor sleep hygiene*: Reliance on alarms, snoozing, drowsiness, reliance on caffeine, lack of attention, forgetfulness, depression, anxiety, irritability, impaired immune system.

*Consequences*: Sleep deprivation can cause various health issues including depression, anxiety, irritability, and frequent illnesses.

**Poor Habits That Impair Sleep**

1. *Drinking Alcohol*: Causes sleep disturbances and poor quality sleep.
2. *Long Daytime Napping*: Can interfere with nighttime sleep, especially in those with sleep issues.
3. *Caffeine and Smoking*: Both act as stimulants; should be avoided 4-6 hours before bedtime.

4. *Lying Awake in Bed*: Can create a negative association with bed; engage in calming activities instead.

5. *Inconsistent Sleep Schedule*: Disrupts circadian rhythm; maintain a regular sleep-wake cycle.

6. *Eating a Large Meal Before Bedtime*: Can cause heartburn and frequent urination.

**Benefits of Good Sleep Hygiene**
- Increased daytime energy
- Improved mood
- Enhanced immune system function
- Reduced stress
- Better cognitive function
- Improved blood glucose control
- Enhanced mental health and productivity

## How To Improve Sleep Through Sleep Hygiene

1. *Have a Sleep Routine*: Stick to a consistent sleep schedule.

2. *Avoid Certain Foods and Beverages*: No caffeine, nicotine, or alcohol 4-6 hours before bed.

3. *Create a Sleep-Promoting Environment*: Keep the bedroom cool, dark, and quiet; invest in comfortable bedding.

4. *Relax Before Bedtime*: Avoid screens, take a warm bath, or engage in calming activities.

5. *Get Up if Not Sleeping*: If unable to sleep after 20 minutes, do a quiet activity until drowsy.

6. *Avoid Sleeping with Pets*: Pets can cause allergies and disturb sleep.

7. *Avoid Late Naps*: Keep naps short and early in the afternoon.

8. *Exercise Regularly*: Improves sleep quality; even 10 minutes of exercise helps.

9. *Avoid Snoozing the Alarm*: Disrupts natural wake-up process; aim to wake up after the first alarm.

**Additional Tips**

- Get natural light exposure in the morning.
- Avoid clock-watching at night.
- Maintain daily activities despite tiredness.
- Avoid eating and intense exercise close to bedtime.
- Stay hydrated but avoid too much fluid before bed.

**Improving Sleep Environment**

- Keep bedroom temperature between 60°F and 70°F.
- Remove noise and light sources; use blackout curtains.
- Keep the bedroom clutter-free.
- Use blue light-blocking glasses or apps, and avoid screens before bed.
- Declutter the bedroom for a relaxing environment.

# CHAPTER 8

# DEALING WITH SETBACKS

## Common Setbacks in the process Of Treating Insomnia With CBT And Solutions

*Initial Comfort and Resistance to Treatment*

Initial Comfort and Resistance to Treatment refers to the common phenomenon where individuals experiencing insomnia may feel comfortable with their familiar sleep patterns and habits, despite their negative impact, and resist changes proposed during Cognitive Behavioral Therapy (CBT). A therapist may works with them to address these resistances, explore underlying beliefs and fears, and gradually introduce new habits to overcome insomnia.

David, a 40-year-old software engineer, has developed a habit of working late into the night to meet deadlines. He feels it's necessary to get things done and believes sleep can wait. His therapist explains how this behavior perpetuates his insomnia and suggests setting boundaries around work hours. David feels initial comfort in his familiar routine and resists changing it, saying, "But I need to get this done, and I can't sleep until it's finished." He experiences a setback in his therapy progress. He finds it difficult to disconnect from work-related tasks and often finds himself checking work emails and taking work calls late into the night. He feels anxious about not meeting deadlines and worries that his work will suffer if he doesn't put in the extra hours and thereby loses more hours of sleep.

How can David deal with this ? Let's say his therapist helps him challenge this thought by asking him to consider alternative scenarios, such as breaking his work into smaller tasks. David will start to see that his belief is not absolute and begins to explore new ways of managing his work. However David might feel discouraged if he keeps reverting to old habits, then he can begin to identify underlying fears and beliefs that drives this habits and begin to reframe his thoughts towards work and productivity and with time and effort he learns to prioritize his tasks, set realistic boundaries with his work hours, and practice self-compassion when he feels overwhelmed. He starts to see that he can be productive and meet his deadlines without sacrificing his sleep and well-being.

## *Lack of Motivation*

Lack of motivation is a common setback in Cognitive Behavioral Therapy for Insomnia (CBT-I). It can manifest in various ways, such as:

- Difficulty initiating or maintaining changes in sleep habits
- Struggling to complete therapy exercises
- Canceling or rescheduling therapy sessions
- Feeling disconnected from the therapy process

Rachel, a 30-year-old marketing specialist, starts CBT-I with enthusiasm but soon finds herself struggling to maintain her new sleep schedule. She starts hitting the snooze button again and stays up late to watch TV. Rachel feels guilty and frustrated, wondering why she can't stick to her goals.

As she experiences these setbacks, Rachel begins to feel like she's failing at therapy. She starts to doubt her ability to change her sleep habits and wonders if she's just not cut out for this. She feels like she's not living up to her own expectations.

*How does Rachel deal with this?*

Rachel needs to explore what's driving her lack of motivation. Careful probing will reveal the source of these setbacks, for example that she might be feeling overwhelmed with work projects and has been using TV as a way to unwind or that she's been comparing herself to others who seem to be making progress faster.

At this point Rachel needs to acknowledge that setbacks are a normal part of the process, she needs to identify and challenge negative thoughts and beliefs (e.g., "I'm a failure if I don't stick to my schedule perfectly") and works with a therapist to develop a more realistic and flexible sleep schedule that takes into account her work demands and relaxation needs and focus on progress, not perfection

With this, Rachel can start to see that it's okay to have days off and that she can get back on track without beating herself up over it, learns to be kinder to herself and to focus on the small wins, and starts to celebrate her successes, no matter how small they may seem. And realizes that progress is not a straight line, but a journey with ups and downs.

By addressing her lack of motivation and developing a more compassionate approach, Rachel is able to overcome her setbacks and continue making progress in her therapy. She learns to prioritize her sleep and her well-being, and she starts to feel more confident and empowered in the process.

***Unrealistic expectations for therapy results***
This occurs when individuals expect immediate or perfect results, or have unrealistic beliefs about what therapy can achieve.

Jack, a 35-year-old entrepreneur, believes that therapy will completely eliminate his insomnia. He's invested time and money into CBT-I and expects a complete cure. However, after a few sessions, he still experiences occasional sleepless nights.

Feeling discouraged and frustrated, Jack starts to doubt the therapy process. He wonders if he's doing something wrong or if CBT-I is just not effective for him. He begins to feel like he's failing at therapy, and his self-doubt and anxiety increase.

*How does Jack resolve this ?*
Jack needs to explore his thoughts and feelings about the setbacks to discover his unrealistic expectations and his fear of not being able to overcome his insomnia.

He needs to understand that setbacks are a normal part of the therapy process, that progress is not always linear, CBT-I aims to manage and improve sleep quality, not eliminate insomnia entirely and it is important to focus on progress, not perfection.

With this new understanding, Jack needs to adjust his expectations and approach and begin practicing self-compassion and acknowledge his efforts, celebrate small successes, like improved sleep quality or reduced anxiety and focus on the skills and strategies he's learning in therapy, also develop a growth mindset, viewing setbacks as opportunities for growth and learning.

By addressing his unrealistic expectations and developing a more realistic and compassionate approach, Jack is able to overcome his setbacks and continue making progress in therapy. He learns to manage his insomnia and improve his overall well-being, and he develops a greater appreciation for the therapy process.

### *Comorbid Conditions*
Comorbid conditions refer to the presence of one or more additional mental health or medical conditions alongside insomnia. These conditions

can impact the effectiveness of Cognitive Behavioral Therapy for Insomnia (CBT-I) and lead to setbacks.

Sarah, a 25-year-old graduate student, experiences insomnia and generalized anxiety disorder (GAD). She starts CBT-I with enthusiasm, but soon finds herself struggling to practice relaxation techniques and sleep schedule changes. Her anxiety overwhelms her, making it difficult to calm her mind and body before sleep.

Feeling frustrated and defeated, Sarah starts to doubt her ability to overcome her insomnia. She wonders if she's just not cut out for CBT-I or if her anxiety is too severe. She begins to feel like she's failing at therapy, and her self-doubt and anxiety increase.

*How does Sarah deal with this ?*
Sarah needs to understand this that:
- Setbacks are a normal part of the therapy process

- Anxiety is a common comorbid condition with insomnia, and it's not a failure on her part
- CBT-I can be adapted to address both insomnia and anxiety
- She's not alone in her struggles, and many people have overcome similar challenges

With this new understanding, Sarah needs to begin to adjust her approach and take these steps:

- Practice anxiety-reducing techniques, such as deep breathing and progressive muscle relaxation
- Break down large goals into smaller, manageable tasks
- Celebrate small successes, like practicing relaxation techniques for a few minutes each day
- Work with her therapist to develop a more realistic and compassionate mindset

By addressing her co-morbid anxiety and developing a more adaptive approach, Sarah starts to notice improvements in her sleep and overall well-being. She realizes that setbacks are not failures, but opportunities for growth and learning. She becomes more confident in her ability to manage her anxiety and insomnia, and she starts to see the value in the therapy process.

## *Environmental and lifestyle factors*

Environmental and lifestyle factors refer to the external circumstances and daily habits that can impact sleep quality and insomnia treatment. These factors can lead to setbacks during Cognitive Behavioral Therapy for Insomnia (CBT-I) if not addressed.

Emily, a 30-year-old marketing specialist, experiences insomnia and starts CBT-I. She's motivated to overcome her sleep struggles, but her work schedule changes, requiring her to work late nights and travel frequently. She's constantly in different time zones, making it challenging to maintain a consistent sleep schedule.

As Emily struggles to adapt to her new schedule, she faces environmental factors that disrupt her sleep. Her hotel rooms are often noisy, and the beds are uncomfortable. She starts to feel like she's taking steps backward in her therapy progress.

Feeling frustrated and overwhelmed, Emily begins to doubt her ability to overcome her insomnia. She wonders if she's just not cut out for this therapy thing or if her lifestyle is too chaotic. She starts to feel like she's failing at therapy, and her self-doubt and anxiety increase.

*What does Emily need to do to solve this ?*

Emily needs to face her fears and doubts and challenge them with questions and alternative options. She needs to understand setbacks are a normal part of the therapy process and changes are bound to happen in life. And even though environmental factors can impact sleep, there are ways to adapt, also she is not alone in her struggles, many people have overcome similar challenges.

With this new understanding, Emily can start to adjust her approach and begin to:

- Prioritize sleep and relaxation techniques despite her busy schedule
- Use earplugs and eye masks to create a sleep-conducive environment in her hotel rooms
- Practice relaxation techniques, like deep breathing and progressive muscle relaxation, to help her cope with noise and discomfort
- Work with her therapist to develop a more realistic and compassionate mindset

By addressing her environmental factors and developing a more adaptive approach to her lifestyle. Emily is able to overcome her setbacks and continue making progress in CBT-I. She learns to manage her sleep and anxiety, even in challenging environments, and she develops a greater appreciation for the therapy process.

## How To Get Back On Track After A Setback

Here is a summary of some practical steps to take to get back on track after experiencing a setback in CBT-I therapy

***Acknowledge and accept the setback***: Recognize that setbacks are a normal part of the therapy process. Avoid self-criticism and blame

***Identify the trigger***: Reflect on the events or circumstances that led to the setback. Identify any patterns or common triggers

***Re-establish a consistent sleep schedule***: Go back to your regular sleep schedule and routine. Avoid napping or sleeping in late

***Practice relaxation techniques***: Engage in relaxation techniques like deep breathing, progressive muscle relaxation, or mindfulness meditation. Use these techniques to manage stress and anxiety

***Review and adjust your therapy plan***: Discuss the setback with your therapist. Adjust your therapy plan to address the trigger and prevent future setbacks.

***Focus on progress, not perfection***: Remember that progress is not always linear. Celebrate small victories and acknowledge progress made so far.

***Seek support***: Reach out to your therapist or support system for guidance and encouragement. Share your experiences and feelings with others to gain perspective.

***Learn from the setback***: Reflect on what you could have done differently. Use the setback as an opportunity to learn and grow.

***Take small steps***: Break down large goals into smaller, manageable tasks. Focus on making progress one step at a time.

***Practice self-compassion***: Treat yourself with kindness and understanding. Remember that setbacks are a normal part of the therapy process.

***SUMMARY***

**Common Setbacks in Treating Insomnia with CBT and Solutions**

1. Initial Comfort and Resistance to Treatment
Individuals may feel comfortable with familiar sleep habits despite negative impacts.
*Example*: David resists changing late-night work habits despite therapy suggestions.
*Solution*: Challenge thoughts, break tasks into smaller pieces, identify underlying fears, reframe thoughts, and gradually adopt new habits.

2. Lack of Motivation
Difficulty initiating/maintaining changes, completing therapy exercises, attending sessions.
*Example*: Rachel struggles to maintain a sleep schedule, feels guilty and frustrated.
*Solution*: Explore causes of low motivation, acknowledge setbacks as normal, adjust sleep

schedule, focus on progress, practice self-compassion.

3. Unrealistic Expectations for Therapy Results

Expecting immediate or perfect results from therapy.

*Example*: Jack expects complete elimination of insomnia and feels discouraged by occasional sleepless nights.

*Solution*: Adjust expectations, understand setbacks are normal, focus on progress, practice self-compassion, celebrate small successes, adopt a growth mindset.

4. Comorbid Conditions

Presence of additional mental health or medical conditions impacting insomnia treatment.

*Example*: Sarah struggles with both insomnia and generalized anxiety disorder (GAD).

*Solution*: Adapt CBT-I to address both conditions, practice anxiety-reducing techniques, break goals into smaller tasks, celebrate small successes, develop a compassionate mindset.

5. Environmental and Lifestyle Factors

External circumstances and daily habits disrupting sleep.

*Example*: Emily's work schedule changes and frequent travel make maintaining sleep consistency difficult.

*Solution*: Prioritize sleep, use earplugs/eye masks, practice relaxation techniques, adjust therapy plan, maintain a realistic and compassionate approach.

**How to Get Back on Track After a Setback**

1. Acknowledge and Accept the Setback: Recognize setbacks as a normal part of therapy without self-criticism.

2. Identify the Trigger: Reflect on events or circumstances that led to the setback and identify patterns.

3. Re-establish a Consistent Sleep Schedule: Return to your regular sleep routine, avoiding naps and sleeping in late.

4. Practice Relaxation Techniques: Use deep breathing, progressive muscle relaxation, or mindfulness to manage stress and anxiety.

5. Review and Adjust Your Therapy Plan: Discuss the setback with your therapist and adjust your plan accordingly.

6. Focus on Progress, Not Perfection: Celebrate small victories and acknowledge progress, recognizing that it's not always linear.

7. Seek Support: Reach out to your therapist or support system for guidance and encouragement.

8. Learn from the Setback: Reflect on what could have been done differently and use the experience for growth.

9. Take Small Steps: Break down large goals into smaller, manageable tasks and focus on incremental progress.

10. Practice Self-compassion: Treat yourself with kindness, understanding that setbacks are a normal part of the process.

# CHAPTER 9

# CONCLUSION

## Recap Of CBT For Insomnia

### Chapter 1: Understanding Insomnia

**Definition and Types**

*Insomnia*: Difficulty in falling asleep, staying asleep, or achieving restful sleep. Defined by AASM as persistent difficulty with sleep initiation, duration, consolidation, or quality.

*Short-term insomnia*: Caused by stress, lasting days to weeks.

*Chronic insomnia*: Lasts at least three nights a week for a minimum of three months, often exacerbated by certain behaviors.

**Types of insomnia:**

*Sleep-onset insomnia*: Difficulty falling asleep.

*Sleep maintenance insomnia*: Difficulty staying asleep.

*Sleep dissatisfaction*: Feeling unrefreshed after sleep.

Medical and psychological comorbidities can contribute to insomnia.

Complex forms:

*Idiopathic insomnia*: No known cause, often lifelong.

*Paradoxical insomnia*: Perception of poor sleep despite normal sleep parameters.

*Psychophysiological insomnia*: Chronic hyperarousal affecting sleep.

**Causes and Risk Factors**

*Psychological conditions*: Anxiety, OCD, PTSD, schizophrenia.

*Lifestyle factors*: Poor sleep hygiene, irregular sleep schedules, substance use.

Risk factors: Age, family history, shift work, environmental disruptions, lifestyle choices.

## Three-factor model (3P)

*Predisposing factors*: Characteristics increasing susceptibility.

*Precipitating factors*: Environmental stressors triggering insomnia.

*Perpetuating factors*: Behaviors and thoughts maintaining insomnia.

## Effects on Health and Well-Being

Difficulties falling asleep, staying asleep, or waking up too early.

*Long-term health risks*: Obesity, diabetes, high blood pressure, heart failure.

Immune system disruption and reduced ability to fight illness.

Impaired blood sugar metabolism, increasing diabetes risk.

*Cognitive impairments*: Memory, concentration, decision-making issues.

Increased stress and risk of mood disorders.
Chronic fatigue impacting daily life.
Reduced life expectancy.

## Chapter 2: CBT for Insomnia

### Overview of CBT-I
Cognitive Behavioral Therapy for Insomnia (CBT-I): Effective non-pharmacological treatment with minimal side effects. Preferred over medication for long-term improvements.

### Components of CBT-I
Sensory control, sleep restriction, cognitive restructuring.
Aims to address dysregulated sleep drive, sleep-related anxiety, and sleep-interfering behaviors.
Typically involves 4-8 sessions of 30-60 minutes.
Drawbacks: Initial reduction in sleep time, benefits not seen until 3-4 weeks into therapy.

Advantages over medication: Fewer adverse effects, addresses root causes of insomnia.

## Components of CBT-I

*Cognitive Therapy*: Identifies and changes unhealthy thoughts and attitudes about sleep.

*Stimulus Control*: Reinforces the bed-sleep association and avoids stimulating activities in bed.

*Sleep Restriction*: Limits time in bed to improve sleep drive and efficiency.

*Sleep Hygiene*: Provides advice on environmental, physiological, and behavioral factors for good sleep.

*Relaxation Methods*: Techniques to reduce cognitive alertness and physical tension (e.g., meditation, mindfulness).

## Evidence of CBT-I Effectiveness

Improves sleep quality, insomnia severity, mood, anxiety, and daily function.

Meta-analyses: Effective for both children and adults, including computerized and group-based formats.

Long-lasting effects compared to hypnotics, with fewer side effects. More effective than hypnotics for chronic insomnia, with benefits lasting up to 6 months. CBT-I recommended as first-line treatment for chronic insomnia.

*Studies*: Significant improvements in sleep efficiency, onset delay, and reduced waking time.

Combination with medication may yield short-term benefits, but CBT-I alone maintains long-term gains. Meta-analysis: Average treatment effect size of 1.0 to 1.2, with improvements lasting up to 24 months. Effective for patients with comorbid medical and behavioral disorders.

## Chapter 3: Stimulus Control Therapy (SCT)

### Explanation of SCT

*Purpose*: Strengthen sleep cues associated with bed/bedroom and establish regular sleep-wake patterns.

*Aim*: Relearn positive connections between bed/bedroom and sleep through methods such as:
Going to bed only when tired.
Establishing a regular wake-up time.
Leaving bed/bedroom after extended wakefulness.
Avoiding non-sleep activities in bed/bedroom.
Not taking naps.

*Theory*: Based on behavioral conditioning; addresses maladaptive conditioning patterns in insomnia patients.

### Steps to Implement SCT

1. Lying down only when sleepy: Enhances awareness of the body's sleep signals. Gradual goal to develop regular sleep habits.

2. Avoiding bed for activities other than sleep/sex: Reinforces sleep cues associated with the bed. Prevent conditioning bed as a place for wakefulness.

3. Getting out of bed if unable to sleep within 15-20 minutes: Reduces frustration associated with wakefulness in bed. Encourages engaging in relaxing activities before returning to bed.

4. Waking up at the same time every day: Strengthens circadian rhythm. Minimizes disruption of sleep-wake patterns.

5. Avoiding napping: Enhances sleep drive for the night. Reinforces night-time sleep cues.

**Common Strategies and Principles**

1. *Waking up at a certain time*: Consistency in wake-up times improves sleep signals. Regular sleep patterns reduce daytime fatigue and drowsiness.

2. *Going to bed only when sleepy*: Focus on internal sleep signals rather than clock time. Gradually develop awareness of tiredness.

3. *Getting out of bed when not ready to sleep*: Limits wakefulness in bed. Engaging in relaxing activities until feeling sleepy.

4. *Using bedroom solely for sleeping*: Avoid stimulating activities in bed/bedroom. Reinforces bedroom as a sleep cue.

5. *Avoiding naps during the day*: Increases likelihood of falling asleep quickly at night. Reinforces sleep pattern regularity.

**Common Obstacles and Solutions**

1. *Time spent in bed before getting out*: Move the clock out of view to avoid clock-watching. Focus on feelings of frustration as cue to get out of bed. Do not stay in bed for extended periods if unable to sleep.

2. *Permissible activities and duration before returning to bed*: Stay out of bed long enough to feel sleepy. Engage in quiet, enjoyable activities with dim lighting. Avoid computer activities and bright lights.

3. *Waking up early*: Return to bed if 45 minutes or more remain until wake-up time. Even small amounts of additional sleep improve alertness and reduce fatigue.

**Notes**

Self-help nature: Requires active participation and adherence to the treatment plan.

Partner collaboration: Discuss strategies with partners to ensure cooperation.

Winter adjustments: Use warm robes and heated rooms to encourage leaving bed during cold weather.

## Chapter 4: Sleep Restriction Therapy (SRT)

**Concept and Benefits of SRT**

Stress or poor sleep habits can lead to insomnia, causing daytime fatigue and a misconception that more time in bed is needed. More time in bed often results in more awake time, leading to anxiety and worsening sleep quality. SRT limits time in bed to improve sleep quality, increase deep sleep, reduce sleep latency, and decrease nighttime awakenings.

SRT is a part of Cognitive Behavioral Therapy for Insomnia (CBT-I) and has been in use for over 30 years.

**Indications for SRT**

SRT is recommended for sleep efficiency below 85% (or 80% in older adults).

SRT can benefit individuals with inconsistent sleep patterns even if their overall sleep efficiency is above 85%.

**Steps to Implement SRT**

1. *Evaluate Sleep Patterns*: Use a sleep diary to determine average sleep length, wake-up time, and best sleep period.
2. *Set Time in Bed (TIB)*: Initially, TIB is set to average sleep length (minimum of 5 hours), with a fixed wake-up time.
3. *Weekly Adjustment*: Adjust TIB based on sleep efficiency (SE) measured weekly:
   - SE ≥90%: Increase TIB by 15-30 minutes.

  - SE 85-90%: Keep TIB unchanged.

  - SE <85%: Decrease TIB by 15-30 minutes.

4. *Consistency*: Maintain strict bedtime and wake-up times, avoid naps, and adhere to the schedule to build sleep pressure.

5. *Monitor and Adjust*: Continue adjustments until optimal sleep duration and quality are achieved.

## Common Obstacles and Solutions

*Scheduled Bedtime*: Flexibility is allowed, but the wake-up time must be adhered to.

*Compliance*: Collaborate with a sleep doctor to tailor the schedule.

*Managing Side Effects*: Start with a slightly longer TIB if experiencing severe side effects.

*Staying Alert*: Use bright lights, exercise, and avoid stimulants.

## Precautions

SRT is not suitable for individuals requiring constant alertness, or those with certain medical conditions like epilepsy or sleep-disordered breathing. It is less effective for individuals with naturally compact sleep or those staying in bed "completely awake."

By following these steps and guidelines, SRT aims to consolidate sleep, improve sleep quality, and reduce daytime fatigue.

## Chapter 5: Relaxation Techniques

### Overview of Relaxation Techniques

Relaxation therapy, historically utilized to treat insomnia, addresses physiological and cognitive arousal in sleep-related performance anxiety and nighttime arousal. Its goal is to reduce or eliminate sleep-disrupting factors such as muscular tension and racing thoughts. Techniques include progressive muscle relaxation, autogenic training, biofeedback-assisted relaxation, guided imagery, deep breathing exercises, physical activity, meditation, and hypnosis. This chapter provides an overview of these techniques and instructions on how to practice them.

*Progressive Muscle Relaxation*
Overview: Also known as Jacobson's Relaxation, this method involves tightening and then releasing different muscle groups to promote relaxation.

Steps:
1. Preparation: Select a distraction-free room and sit or lie comfortably.
2. Feet: Contract foot muscles for 5 seconds, release for 10 seconds.
3. Lower Legs: Contract and release muscles in the lower legs.
4. Hips and Buttocks: Repeat the process.
5. Torso: Focus on stomach and chest muscles.
6. Shoulders: Contract and release shoulder muscles.
7. Face: Contract facial muscles by pressing eyes shut, then release.

*Autogenic Training*
Overview: This technique promotes psychological and physical calm by controlling breathing and responding to verbal commands to focus on body sensations like warmth and heaviness.

How To Do It:
1. Setup: Find a quiet, comfortable place to relax.
2. Breath Focus: Begin with calm, even breathing.
3. Body Focus: Sequentially focus on different body parts, repeating calming statements.
4. Heartbeat Focus: Inhale deeply, affirm a calm heartbeat, and relax.

*Biofeedback-Assisted Relaxation*
Overview: Uses electrical instruments to monitor body processes like skin temperature, heart rate, and muscle tension to help control these areas.

How It Works:
1. Monitoring: Sensors are attached to the body, providing data on physiological processes.

2. Feedback: Use the data to adjust and relax specific body areas.

*Guided Imagery Training*
Overview: Involves visualizing peaceful settings to replace negative or stressful feelings with positive and calming experiences.

Steps:
1. Setup: Sit or lie down comfortably in a distraction-free area.
2. Visualization: Imagine a tranquil environment using all five senses.
3. Relaxation: Continue the visualization while taking deep breaths.

*Deep Breathing Exercises*
Overview: Linked to slower heart rates and lower blood pressure, deep breathing, or belly breathing, promotes calmness.

Box Breathing Technique:

1. Inhale: Breathe in through your nose for 2-4 seconds.
2. Hold: Hold your breath for 2-4 seconds.
3. Exhale: Breathe out for 2-4 seconds.
4. Hold: Hold your breath again for 2-4 seconds.
5. Repeat: Continue as needed.

*Physical Activity*

Overview: Exercise promotes the release of endorphins, enhancing sleep. Activities like tai chi, qigong, and yoga incorporate mindfulness and promote relaxation.

*Meditation*

Overview: Meditation calms the mind and body, promoting inner peace and alleviating insomnia by reducing stress and anxiety.

Benefits:
- Increases melatonin and serotonin levels.
- Reduces heart rate and blood pressure.

- Engages brain areas regulating sleep.

*Hypnosis*

Overview: Sleep hypnosis can assist those with insomnia by promoting relaxation and reducing anxiety. It is often more effective when combined with other psychological therapies.

How It Works:

Preparation: Relaxation and entering a trance-like state.

Goals: Setting goals with a hypnotherapist and following their guidance.

Benefits of Relaxation Techniques

Relaxation techniques can help manage various health issues, including labor pain, heart disease, chemotherapy-related nausea, chronic pain, and temporomandibular joint pain.

## Instructions for Practicing Relaxation Techniques

*Breathing Techniques: 4-7-8 Breathing*

1. Preparation: Find a comfortable spot, sit or lie down, and maintain good posture.
2. Breath Cycle:
   - Exhale completely through your mouth.
   - Inhale quietly through your nose for 4 seconds.
   - Hold your breath for 7 seconds.
   - Exhale completely through your mouth for 8 seconds.
3. Repeat: Continue for four full breaths.

*Autogenic Training:*

1. Setup: Choose a quiet place, sit or lie comfortably, remove distractions.
2. Breathing: Start with calm, even breathing.
3. Body Focus: Sequentially focus on different body parts, repeating calming statements.

*Guided Imagery*:
1. Setup: Sit or lie down comfortably in a quiet place.
2. Visualization: Imagine a peaceful scene using all senses.
3. Relaxation: Continue visualization with deep breaths.

*Progressive Muscle Relaxation*:
1. Preparation: Lay or sit down, relax your body.
2. Muscle Tensing and Relaxing: Focus on one muscle group at a time, tensing for 5 seconds, then relaxing for 10-20 seconds.

*Biofeedback Therapy*:
1. Monitoring: Use sensors to monitor physiological processes.
2. Adjustments: Use feedback to learn how to control and relax specific body areas.

*Meditation*:
1. Setup: Find a quiet place, sit or lie down.
2. Breathing: Take calm, deep breaths.
3. Focus: Concentrate on your breathing and let go of distracting thoughts.

Incorporating these relaxation techniques into your daily routine can help manage stress and improve sleep quality. Start with one or two techniques and practice them consistently to see the best results.

## Chapter 6: Cognitive Therapy and Restructuring

**Explanation of Cognitive Therapy**
Aims to change sleep-related cognitions (beliefs, attitudes, expectancies) contributing to insomnia. Focuses on examining negative feelings that interfere with sleep. Guides individuals in identifying and reframing unhelpful sleep-related beliefs.

## Identifying and Challenging Negative Thoughts and Beliefs about Sleep

*Specific therapeutic objectives*:

Unreasonable expectations regarding sleep ("I must get 8 hours every night").

Incorrect assumptions about insomnia causes ("It's entirely due to a biochemical imbalance").

Excessive stress about sleep loss consequences ("Insomnia will have serious health effects").

Misunderstandings about sleep habits ("If I try harder, I'll fall asleep").

*Techniques used*:

Socratic questioning, collaborative empiricism, and guided discovery.

Identifying automatic beliefs, linking cognitions to emotions and behaviors, and replacing distorted thoughts with accurate interpretations.

*Self-Monitoring*

Important for recognizing automatic thinking patterns.

Can be achieved through Socratic questioning and using an automatic thoughts record form.

*Example of Automatic Thoughts Record Form*

Situation: Specify date and time.

Automatic Thoughts: What was going through your mind?

Emotions: Rate intensity (1–100%).

*Cognitive Restructuring Techniques*

Self-Monitoring: Recognize and record counterproductive thoughts.

Challenging Assumptions: Use Socratic questioning to investigate and challenge negative thoughts.

Gathering Evidence: Keep a journal or sleep diary to record events, emotions, and thoughts.

Cost-Benefit Evaluation: Assess the practical and emotional costs and benefits of clinging to negative thoughts.

Generating Alternatives: Develop logical replacements for cognitive distortions and create empowering affirmations.

*Positive Affirmations*

Replace negative beliefs with positive, constructive statements.

Examples:
 - "I will sleep soundly all through the night."
 - "My bedroom is a place of relaxation and deep sleep."
 - "I will get up as soon as my alarm goes off and feel fresh and alert."
 - Tailor affirmations to your specific situation and keep them in the present tense.

Benefits of Affirmations
- Reduce stress and anxiety.
- Improve sleep quality.
- Promote a consistent pre-bedtime routine.

## Importance of Good Sleep Hygiene

*Signs of poor sleep hygiene*: Reliance on alarms, snoozing, drowsiness, reliance on caffeine, lack of attention, forgetfulness, depression, anxiety, irritability, impaired immune system.

*Consequences*: Sleep deprivation can cause various health issues including depression, anxiety, irritability, and frequent illnesses.

## Poor Habits That Impair Sleep

1. *Drinking Alcohol*: Causes sleep disturbances and poor quality sleep.
2. *Long Daytime Napping*: Can interfere with nighttime sleep, especially in those with sleep issues.
3. *Caffeine and Smoking*: Both act as stimulants; should be avoided 4-6 hours before bedtime.
4. *Lying Awake in Bed*: Can create a negative association with bed; engage in calming activities instead.
5. *Inconsistent Sleep Schedule*: Disrupts circadian rhythm; maintain a regular sleep-wake cycle.

6. *Eating a Large Meal Before Bedtime*: Can cause heartburn and frequent urination.

Benefits of Good Sleep Hygiene
- Increased daytime energy
- Improved mood
- Enhanced immune system function
- Reduced stress
- Better cognitive function
- Improved blood glucose control
- Enhanced mental health and productivity

**How To Improve Sleep Through Sleep Hygiene**

1. *Have a Sleep Routine*: Stick to a consistent sleep schedule.
2. *Avoid Certain Foods and Beverages*: No caffeine, nicotine, or alcohol 4-6 hours before bed.
3. *Create a Sleep-Promoting Environment*: Keep the bedroom cool, dark, and quiet; invest in comfortable bedding.

4. *Relax Before Bedtime*: Avoid screens, take a warm bath, or engage in calming activities.

5. *Get Up if Not Sleeping*: If unable to sleep after 20 minutes, do a quiet activity until drowsy.

6. *Avoid Sleeping with Pets*: Pets can cause allergies and disturb sleep.

7. *Avoid Late Naps*: Keep naps short and early in the afternoon.

8. *Exercise Regularly*: Improves sleep quality; even 10 minutes of exercise helps.

9. *Avoid Snoozing the Alarm*: Disrupts natural wake-up process; aim to wake up after the first alarm.

**Additional Tips**

- Get natural light exposure in the morning.
- Avoid clock-watching at night.
- Maintain daily activities despite tiredness.
- Avoid eating and intense exercise close to bedtime.
- Stay hydrated but avoid too much fluid before bed.

**Improving Sleep Environment**

- Keep bedroom temperature between 60°F and 70°F.
- Remove noise and light sources; use blackout curtains.
- Keep the bedroom clutter-free.
- Use blue light-blocking glasses or apps, and avoid screens before bed.
- Declutter the bedroom for a relaxing environment.

**Common Setbacks in Treating Insomnia with CBT and Solutions**

1. *Initial Comfort and Resistance to Treatment*: Individuals may feel comfortable with familiar sleep habits despite negative impacts.

Example: David resists changing late-night work habits despite therapy suggestions.

Solution: Challenge thoughts, break tasks into smaller pieces, identify underlying fears, reframe thoughts, and gradually adopt new habits.

2. *Lack of Motivation*: Difficulty initiating/maintaining changes, completing therapy exercises, attending sessions.

Example: Rachel struggles to maintain a sleep schedule, feels guilty and frustrated.

Solution: Explore causes of low motivation, acknowledge setbacks as normal, adjust sleep schedule, focus on progress, practice self-compassion.

3. *Unrealistic Expectations for Therapy Results*: Expecting immediate or perfect results from therapy.

Example: Jack expects complete elimination of insomnia and feels discouraged by occasional sleepless nights.

Solution: Adjust expectations, understand setbacks are normal, focus on progress, practice self-compassion, celebrate small successes, adopt a growth mindset.

4. *Comorbid Conditions*: Presence of additional mental health or medical conditions impacting insomnia treatment.

Example: Sarah struggles with both insomnia and generalized anxiety disorder (GAD).

Solution: Adapt CBT-I to address both conditions, practice anxiety-reducing techniques, break goals into smaller tasks, celebrate small successes, develop a compassionate mindset.

5. *Environmental and Lifestyle Factors*: External circumstances and daily habits disrupting sleep.

Example: Emily's work schedule changes and frequent travel make maintaining sleep consistency difficult.

Solution: Prioritize sleep, use earplugs/eye masks, practice relaxation techniques, adjust therapy plan, maintain a realistic and compassionate approach.

**How to Get Back on Track After a Setback**

1. *Acknowledge and Accept the Setback*: Recognize setbacks as a normal part of therapy without self-criticism.

2. *Identify the Trigger*: Reflect on events or circumstances that led to the setback and identify patterns.

3. *Re-establish a Consistent Sleep Schedule*: Return to your regular sleep routine, avoiding naps and sleeping in late.

4. *Practice Relaxation Techniques*: Use deep breathing, progressive muscle relaxation, or mindfulness to manage stress and anxiety.

5. *Review and Adjust Your Therapy Plan*: Discuss the setback with your therapist and adjust your plan accordingly.

6. *Focus on Progress, Not Perfection*: Celebrate small victories and acknowledge progress, recognizing that it's not always linear.

7. *Seek Support*: Reach out to your therapist or support system for guidance and encouragement.

8. Learn from the Setback: Reflect on what could have been done differently and use the experience for growth.

9. *Take Small Steps*: Break down large goals into smaller, manageable tasks and focus on incremental progress.

10. *Practice Self-compassion*: Treat yourself with kindness, understanding that setbacks are a normal part of the process.

## Encouragement And Final Thoughts

The quest to overcome insomnia calls for perseverance, self-compassion, and patience. You have gained invaluable knowledge and useful tools from each chapter to aid you on your journey. Recall that even while progress could seem sluggish at times, each step you take will get you closer to greater and better sleep and overall well being.

Remain dedicated to your sleep health and don't be afraid to ask friends, family, or medical experts for assistance. You are capable of changing for the better and getting deep, rejuvenating sleep. Continue on your path filled with optimism and confidence.

# Sleep Diary

Instructions for using a sleep diary to track progress and identify patterns

1. Make a sleep schedule. Write out the time you intend to go to sleep (bedtime) and the time you intend to wake up (rise time) and follow the schedule for a week
2. Record the dates to mark your schedule
3. After you wake up note your sleep duration and sleep efficiency
4. To get your accurate sleep duration, determine the hours and minutes between your sleep onset time (the time you dozed off) to the time you woke up, remove the duration of nighttime awakenings from it. Then you get your sleep duration.

5. To get sleep efficiency, you divide your sleep duration by total time in bed and multiply by 100%

   S.E = sleep duration/TIB x 100%
6. Note how you got awakened whether by an alarm, a disturbance or spontaneously.

# Template for a sleep diary

Day: _____        Sleep Duration: _____

Date: _____       Sleep Efficiency: _____


How did you woke up in the morning: ____


How did you felt when you woke up this morning: _____


Sleep schedule

| Bedtime  | |
|----------|--|
| Risetime | |

# Questionnaire

Fill after you wake up

| | |
|---|---|
| What time did you go to bed | |
| How many nighttime awakenings did you have | |
| What woke you up in the night | |
| How long did your nighttime awakenings last | |
| What time did you finally woke up | |
| What time do you get out of bed | |
| What is your estimated duration of sleep | |

Fill before you sleep

| How stressful was your day | |
|---|---|
| Did you nap during the day | |
| How many times did you nap | |
| What (is) are duration of your nap(s) | |
| Any alcohol or caffeine intake if yes, when | |
| Any medication intake if yes when | |
| Any Exercises performed during the day if yes when | |
| Activities engaged in before bedtime | |

# Glossary of Terms

Definitions of key terms used in the book

**Actigraphy**: A non-invasive method of monitoring movement and sleep patterns.
**Blue Light**: High-energy visible light emitted by electronic devices that can
interfere with sleep.
**Circadian Rhythm**: The internal biological clock regulating sleep-wake cycles.
**Comorbid Conditions**: Co-occurring health conditions that can impact sleep.
**Comorbid**: Co-occurring health conditions.
**Daytime Fatigue**: Feeling tired or sluggish during the day.
**Hypnotics**: Medications used to induce sleep.
**Idiopathic**: A term used to describe a condition with no known cause.
**Inflammation**: A bodily response to injury or infection that can impact sleep.

**Insomnia**: Difficulty initiating or maintaining sleep.

**Maladaptive**: A term used to describe harmful or unhelpful behaviors.

**Mood Disturbances**: Changes in emotional state, such as irritability or anxiety.

**Naps**: Short periods of sleep taken during the day.

**Paradoxical**: A term used to describe a condition that contradicts expectations.

**Placebo**: A dummy treatment with no active effects.

**Polysomnography (PSG)**: A comprehensive sleep study that records various physiological activities.

**Power Naps**: Short, refreshing naps taken during the day.l

**Schizophrenia**: A mental health condition characterized by hallucinations and delusions.

**Sleep Apnea**: A condition characterized by pauses in breathing during sleep.

**Sleep Architecture**: The structure and organization of sleep stages throughout the night.
**Sleep Consolidation**: The process of entering deeper sleep stages and staying asleep.
**Sleep Cues**: External factors that trigger sleepiness or wakefulness.
**Sleep Cycle**: The stages of sleep and wakefulness that occur throughout the day.
**Sleep Deprivation**: Not getting enough sleep or having sleep disrupted.
**Sleep Diary**: A record of sleep patterns and habits kept by an individual.
**Sleep Diary**: A record of sleep patterns and habits kept by an individual.
**Sleep Disorder**: Any condition that affects sleep quality, duration, or timing.
**Sleep Disruption**: Any disturbance to normal sleep patterns.
**Sleep Disturbances**: Any disruptions or disruptions to normal sleep patterns.
**Sleep Duration**: The length of time spent

sleeping.

**Sleep Efficiency**: The percentage of time spent asleep while in bed.

**Sleep Effort**: The amount of effort put into falling asleep or staying asleep.

**Sleep Environment**: The external factors affecting sleep, such as light, noise, and temperature.

**Sleep Habits**: Regular patterns of sleep behavior.

**Sleep Initiation**: The process of falling asleep.

**Sleep Latency**: The time it takes to fall asleep after going to bed.

**Sleep Medications**: Drugs used to treat sleep disorders.

**Sleep Pattern**: The regular habits and rhythms of sleep.

**Sleep Patterns**: The regular habits and rhythms of sleep.

**Sleep Pressure**: The build-up of the need for sleep.

**Sleep Quality**: A measure of how well sleep is restoring and refreshing.

**Sleep Questionnaires**: Surveys used to assess sleep quality and habits.

**Sleep Record**: A documentation of sleep patterns and habits.

**Sleep Stages**: The different phases of sleep, including REM and non-REM sleep.

**Stimulus Dyscontrol**: Difficulty regulating responses to external stimuli.

**Stress**: A state of mental or emotional tension that can affect sleep.

www.ingramcontent.com/pod-product-compliance
Lightning Source LLC
Chambersburg PA
CBHW071914210526
45479CB00002B/413